ENDOCRINE
REPLACEMENT THERAPY

NEW APPROACHES

*Based on a conference organised by the
Royal College of Physicians of London*

Edited by

James Ahlquist

Consultant Physician and Endocrinologist

John Wass

Consultant Physician

ROYAL COLLEGE OF PHYSICIANS OF LONDON
1996

Royal College of Physicians of London
11 St Andrews Place, London NW1 4LE

Registered Charity No. 210508

Copyright © 1996 Royal College of Physicians of London
ISBN 1 86016 0522

Typeset by Dan-Set Graphics, Telford, Shropshire
Printed in Great Britain by APW, Newport, Shropshire

Preface

Replacing hormone deficiency states is now known to be more complex than was appreciated in the past. New issues are emerging, for example, who should receive replacement therapy, which hormones should be replaced, just what are the benefits of oestrogen, should men be given androgen replacement, and where does growth hormone replacement fit in for the clinician in practice? This book addresses these issues, and more. The chapters are based on papers presented at a conference of the Royal College of Physicians, as part of the Interfaces in Medicine series. This is a series of conferences designed to look at medical issues where there are important recent developments of interest to both specialists and generalists.

The book opens with some of the more controversial issues in endocrine replacement. Thyroxine is prescribed to half a million people in the UK every year—but how much should we give? What are the potential harms of too much or too little? Jayne Franklyn reviews the evidence and considers the role of biochemical monitoring of these patients. Eberhard Nieschlag and Hermann Behre look at the developing area of androgen replacement therapy in men. Who should be treated? What methods are available, and how should the treatment be monitored? Growth hormone replacement in adulthood is reviewed by Peter Sönksen. This is a particularly controversial area in which views are rapidly changing. Clinicians are likely to see an increasing use of growth hormone in adults in the future, now that its use as replacement therapy in adults has been licensed. We need to be equipped to deal with the issues of whom to treat, for how long, and how to monitor treatment. Glucocorticoid replacement therapy also comes under the spotlight: Trevor Howlett presents the results of his experience in monitoring replacement, and considers the possible adverse effects of over- and under-treatment.

The second half of the book concentrates on the important issues surrounding sex hormone replacement therapy in women—'HRT'. This section will doubtless be of interest to many readers. Juliet Compston examines the place of HRT in the prevention of osteoporosis, and also gives practical advice on the assessment of osteoporosis, and the place of bone densitometry. David Crook and John Stevenson present an overview of the effects of HRT on serum lipids and lipoproteins, and the ways in which HRT may be used to reduce the risk of cardiovascular disease. What is the evidence that HRT does reduce cardiovascular disease? Tom Meade and Madge Vickers review the evidence, and set it in an appropriate epidemiological context. Finally Margaret Rees considers the practical aspects of HRT, including non-menstrual forms of therapy, and looks at the ways in which the choice of preparation can increase the acceptability of the treatment for the patient.

The field of endocrine replacement therapy is changing fast. Even since the conference was held, new therapies that were discussed at the meeting have become available for general clinical use. We present this volume in the hope that it will be useful to all involved in the care of the post-menopausal woman or those patients with endocrine deficiency states, whether in hospital practice or in primary care.

October 1996

JAMES AHLQUIST
JOHN WASS
Editors

Contributors

James AO Ahlquist MB MRCP(UK) *Consultant Physician and Endocrinologist, Southend Hospital, Westcliff-on-Sea, Essex SS0 0RY; formerly: Department of Endocrinology, Radcliffe Infirmary, Oxford OX2 6HE*

Hermann M Behre DM *Senior Physician, Institute of Reproductive Medicine, University of Münster, Domagkstr. 11, D-48129 Münster, Germany*

Juliet E Compston MD FRCP FRCPath *Senior Research Associate and Honorary Consultant Physician, Department of Medicine, University of Cambridge Clinical School, Addenbrooke's Hospital, Hills Road, Cambridge CB2 2QQ*

David Crook PhD *Lecturer, Wynn Institute for Metabolic Research, National Heart and Lung Institute, Imperial College of Science, Technology and Medicine, 21 Wellington Road, London NW8 9SQ*

Jayne A Franklyn MD PhD FRCP *Professor of Medicine, Department of Medicine, University of Birmingham, Queen Elizabeth Hospital, Edgbaston, Birmingham B15 2TH*

Trevor A Howlett MD FRCP *Consultant Physician and Endocrinologist, Leicester Royal Infirmary, Leicester LE1 5WW*

Thomas W Meade CBE DM FRCP FRS *Director, MRC Epidemiology and Medical Care Unit, Wolfson Institute of Preventive Medicine, St Bartholomew's and the Royal London School of Medicine and Dentistry, Charterhouse Square, London EC1M 6BQ*

Eberhard Nieschlag DM FRCP *Director, Institute of Reproductive Medicine, University of Münster, Domagkstr. 11, D-48129 Münster, Germany*

Margaret CP Rees MBBS DPhil MRCOG *Honorary Senior Clinical Lecturer in Obstetrics and Gynaecology, John Radcliffe Hospital, Oxford OX3 9DU*

Peter H Sönksen MD FRCP *Professor of Endocrinology, Division of Medicine, Guy's and St Thomas's Medical and Dental School, St Thomas' Hospital, Lambeth Palace Road, London SE1 7EH*

John C Stevenson MBBS FRCP *Director and Senior Lecturer/Honorary Consultant Physician, Wynn Institute for Metabolic Research, National Heart and Lung Institute, Imperial College of Science, Technology and Medicine, 21 Wellington Road, London NW8 9SQ*

Madge Vickers PhD *Senior Scientist, MRC Epidemiology and Medical Care Unit, Wolfson Institute of Preventive Medicine, St Bartholomew's and the Royal London School of Medicine and Dentistry, Charterhouse Square, London EC1M 6BQ*

John AH Wass MD FRCP *Consultant Physician, Department of Endocrinology, Radcliffe Infirmary, Oxford OX2 6HE*

Contents

1 | Thyroid hormone replacement therapy—how much is too much?

Jayne A Franklyn
Professor of Medicine, Department of Medicine,
University of Birmingham, Queen Elizabeth Hospital

Thyroxine is one of the most frequently prescribed of all drugs; it is generally given for the treatment of hypothyroidism. A recent prevalence study in the West Midlands indicates that thyroxine is prescribed for almost 1% of the general population and 4% of those aged over 60.[1] Similar prevalence studies in Sweden have revealed that 1.2% of the population is prescribed thyroxine[2] and in the United States, prescriptions for thyroxine comprise 1% of all those written.[3] In the UK approximately 500,000 prescriptions are issued for thyroxine each year.

Thyroid function tests

Although biochemical tests have an important role in the diagnosis of thyroid disease, the value of biochemical monitoring in patients treated with thyroxine is not clear. Improvements in tests of thyroid function, and specifically development of sensitive assays for thyrotrophin (TSH, thyroid stimulating hormone), which distinguish the low values seen in hyperthyroidism from normal values of euthyroidism, has led to the realisation that such measurements are frequently abnormal in those receiving thyroxine replacement therapy. Our own survey of patients recruited from general practice indicated that 20% have a low serum TSH, providing biochemical evidence of over-treatment, whereas 25% have raised serum TSH, indicating under-treatment.[4] Examination of the relationship between such results and the dose of thyroxine prescribed suggests that such biochemical abnormalities often reflect inappropriate dose prescription. This is particularly a problem where the prescribed dose of thyroxine is too small. There is an additional problem of poor compliance, which is evident in patients with raised serum TSH despite prescription of doses of thyroxine of 200µg a day.[4]

1

Consequences of abnormalities of thyroid function tests in patients prescribed thyroxine

Even though abnormal biochemical results are common in patients taking thyroxine, the pathophysiological significance of these abnormalities is unknown.[5] There is some evidence that overt untreated hypothyroidism is associated with hyperlipidaemia and increased risk of ischaemic heart disease.[6] It is also postulated that mild hypothyroidism, indicated by an elevated serum TSH and associated with inadequate thyroxine treatment, may have similar associated risks. In contrast, overt hyperthyroidism is associated with reduction in bone mineral density and increased risk of osteoporotic fractures and it is postulated that mild biochemical hyperthyroidism, indicated by a modest increase in serum T4 and suppression of serum TSH to below normal, often associated with thyroxine therapy, has similar risks[7] (Table 1).

Thyroxine therapy

Effect on lipids

Studies of the effect of mild hypothyroidism and its treatment with thyroxine on circulating lipids have produced conflicting results.[8]

Table 1. The possible health risks of abnormal levels of serum TSH. Interpretation of TSH values in patients receiving thyroxine replacement therapy, and the possible consequences for long-term health. (See the text for an analysis of the clinical significance of abnormal TSH values in replacement therapy).

Serum TSH value	Biochemical interpretation	Possible health consequences
Low	over-treatment with thyroxine	exacerbation of bone mineral loss and increased fracture risk
		increased risk of development of atrial fibrillation
Normal	appropriate thyroxine replacement	normal quality of life and normal life expectancy
Raised	under-treatment with thyroxine	hypercholesterolaemia and increased cardiovascular risk

Some studies have failed to reveal a relationship between mild hypothyroidism and the levels of circulating cholesterol and triglycerides, or any significant change in lipid levels after correction of an elevated serum TSH by increasing the dose of thyroxine prescribed.[9,10] In contrast, other researchers have reported that thyroxine treatment is associated with a favourable change in circulating lipids, namely an increase in serum high-density lipoprotein (HDL) cholesterol and a reduction in low-density lipoprotein (LDL) cholesterol.[11]

Our own studies have revealed that in patients with mild sub-clinical hypothyroidism (indicated by a rise in serum TSH in the absence of a fall in serum T4), treatment with thyroxine is associated with a reduction in both total and LDL cholesterol in serum.[11] The greatest fall in serum cholesterol was associated with an increase in thyroxine dose to that which suppressed TSH to below normal values (typically 150µg a day), rather than a dose that restored serum TSH to the normal range (typically 100µg a day) (Table 2). Likewise, comparison of cholesterol measurements in patients taking sufficient thyroxine to suppress serum TSH with those in a control group indicates that thyroxine treatment abolishes the age-related rise in total and LDL cholesterol measurements in those aged 55 years and over.[12] These data suggest that correction of mild hypothyroidism (indicated by a raised serum TSH alone) is associated with a potentially beneficial change in circulating lipids; moreover, mild thyroxine excess (indicated by a reduced serum TSH) has a greater beneficial effect on lipids than doses that

Table 2. The effect of thyroxine dose on TSH and cholesterol.
Effects of incremental doses of thyroid hormone replacement (2 weeks at each dose) on serum concentrations of TSH, total cholesterol and LDL cholesterol in patients with subclinical hypothyroidism. *P*: significance of differences across doses of thyroxine replacement. From Franklyn *et al.*[12]

T4 dose (µg/day)	Free T4 (pmol/l)	TSH (mU/l)	Total cholesterol (mmol/l)	LDL cholesterol (mmol/l)
0	10.5±0.3	13.8±1.7	7.39±0.56	5.24±0.54
50	17.0±0.9	4.0±0.7	7.10±0.52	5.07±0.43
100	22.0±1.4	1.1±0.3	7.02±0.52	4.90±0.39
150	27.9±3.2	0.1±0.0	6.60±0.47	4.46±0.33
P	*P*<0.001	*P*<0.001	*P*<0.01	*P*<0.01
Normal range	9–25	0.5–5	3.96–6.96	2.26–5.0

restore TSH to normal. However, clinical outcome studies are required to determine the effects on the risk of cardiovascular disease of a mildly elevated or suppressed serum TSH level in patients receiving thyroxine replacement therapy.

Effect on bone mineral density

It is clear that overt hyperthyroidism is associated with bone loss, which is corrected (at least in part) by effective anti-thyroid therapy. However, the question of whether excess thyroid hormone in patients taking thyroxine who have a modestly elevated serum T4 and a suppressed serum TSH level is similarly associated with bone loss, and risk of osteoporotic fracture remains controversial.[7,8] Several studies have suggested that thyroxine therapy is associated with reductions in bone mineral density at various sites,[13,14] although other studies have failed to demonstrate such an effect.[15] Interpretation of the findings from these reports is complicated by the fact that many studies have included small numbers of patients with varying histories of thyroid disease preceding thyroxine therapy, including some with a past history of thyrotoxicosis.

Our own data suggest that patients receiving thyroxine therapy for hypothyroidism, but with no previous history of thyrotoxicosis, do not have reductions in either femoral or lumbar spine bone mineral density compared with controls; this is the case even if thyroxine has been given in high dose for long periods of time in patients with previous thyroid cancer. Furthermore, in those patients with a past history of thyroid cancer who were treated with doses of thyroxine sufficient to suppress serum TSH levels, we found no significant relationship between measurements of bone mineral density and dose or duration of thyroxine treatment.[16] In contrast, we have shown that post-menopausal females with a previous history of thyrotoxicosis treated with radio-iodine and subsequent thyroxine therapy for hypothyroidism have 5 to 10% reductions in femoral and lumbar spine bone density compared with controls.[17] These observations suggest that oestrogen deficiency associated with bone loss at the time of overt excess of thyroid hormone and subsequent mild excess of thyroxine, due to thyroxine therapy, may together have a detrimental effect on bone metabolism. We have recently shown that in such post-menopausal women with a previous history of thyrotoxicosis, treatment with oestrogen replacement therapy in addition to thyroxine abolishes the reduction in bone mineral density compared with non-oestrogen-treated controls.[18] This suggests that this group of women, who are potentially at increased risk of osteoporotic fracture, might be targetted for hormone replacement therapy (HRT).

Clinical consequences of changes in thyroid status associated with thyroxine therapy

Although there is evidence from the general population that low femoral bone density is a predictor of femoral fracture,[19] it is not clear whether significant reductions in bone mineral density related to thyroid dysfunction and its treatment are associated with an increased fracture risk. The importance of osteoporotic fractures, especially fracture of the femur, is well recognised, and the impact of osteoporosis is a major concern for public health.[20] Studies of morbidity and mortality from osteoporotic fracture in patients with thyroid disease are essential. Enormous concern[5] has arisen from reports suggesting a deleterious effect of thyroxine therapy on bone density, and this has led in turn to a recommendation by the American Thyroid Association that thyroxine doses should be adjusted until serum values of TSH are restored to the normal range.[21] However, it is not known whether such changes in bone density are associated with altered risk of relevant clinical endpoints such as fracture rate.[22,23] There have been only a small number of reported studies addressing this question. One such study, involving 1,180 patients treated with thyroxine, compared those with an undetectable TSH level with those patients whose TSH was detectable but not elevated. No difference was found in the overall fracture rate between the two groups.[24] A further study, involving 160 females with thyroid disease, reported no evidence of increased prevalence of fractures, although there was evidence for fractures earlier in life in those with previous hyperthyroidism.[25] It is notable that a recent large prospective study,[26] examining risk factors for hip fracture in post-menopausal women, demonstrated an apparent increased risk among thyroxine takers, which was abolished when a past history of thyrotoxicosis was taken into account. The same study indicated that previous thyrotoxicosis itself increased the risk of femur fracture by a factor of 1.8 (confidence limits 1.2–2.6),[26] findings in accord with the results of studies of bone mineral density described above.

In addition to the question of whether fracture rate is increased by thyroxine therapy, our finding that thyroxine, given in doses that suppress serum TSH, significantly reduces circulating concentrations of total and LDL cholesterol[12] suggests that thyroxine therapy may actually be beneficial in terms of ischaemic heart disease, in view of unequivocal evidence linking total and LDL cholesterol values to heart disease risk[27]—although this view is speculative. An important prospective study of the over-60s has revealed that a low serum TSH concentration represents a risk factor for the development of atrial fibrillation, trebling the likelihood of developing this arrhythmia over a 10-year period of follow-up.[28] While most of the subjects with a low serum TSH concentration in that study were not taking T4, the findings do highlight a potential adverse cardiovascular influence of mild thyroid hormone excess, which is evident biochemically in many patients taking thyroxine long-term. Again, epidemiological studies are required to investigate the cardiovascular consequences of thyroxine therapy, especially those with a serum TSH below the normal range.

Conclusions

Thyroxine replacement therapy is one of the most common prescribed therapies. Many patients on thyroxine have minor abnormalities in thyroid function tests, but the significance of these is as yet uncertain. The American Thyroid Association has proposed that maintenance of serum TSH within the normal range is an appropriate goal of thyroxine therapy in those beginning treatment; however, in the absence of clear epidemiological evidence of benefit or harm associated with abnormal serum TSH results, the recall of large numbers of patients in the community prescribed thyroxine is not warranted at present.

References

1   Parle JV, Franklyn JA, Sheppard MC. Thyroxine replacement therapy. *Lancet* 1991; **337**: 171.
2   Petersen K, Bengstonn C, Lapidus L, Lindstedt G, Nistrom E. Morbidity, mortality, and quality of life for patients treated with thyroxine. *Arch Int Med* 1990; **150**: 2077–81.
3   Kaufman SC, Gross GP, Kennedy DL. Thyroid hormone use: trends in the United States from 1960 through 1988. *Thyroid* 1991; **1**: 285–91.
4   Parle JV, Franklyn JA, Cross K, Jones S, Sheppard MC. Thyroxine prescription in the community: serum thyroid stimulating hormone level assays as an indicator of undertreatment or overtreatment. *Br J Gen Pract* 1993; **43**: 107–9.
5   Anonymous. Thyroxine replacement therapy: too much of a good thing? *Lancet* 1990; **336**: 1352–3.
6   Franklyn JA, Gammage MD. Thyroid disease effect on cardiovascular function. *Trends in Endocrinology and Metabolism* 1996; **7**: 50–4.
7   Baran DT, Braverman LE. Thyroid hormones and bone mass. *J Clin End Metab* 1991; **72**: 1182–3.

8   Roti ER, Minelli R, Gardini E, Braverman LE. The use and misuse of thyroid hormone. *Endoc Rev* 1993; **14**: 401–23.

9   Ridgway EC, Cooper DS, Walker H, Rodbard D, Maloof F. Peripheral responses to thyroid hormone before and after L-thyroxine therapy in patients with subclinical hypothyroidism. *J Clin Endo Metab* 1981; **53**: 1238–42.

10   Cooper DS, Halpern R, Wood LC, Levin AA, Ridgway EC. L-thyroxine therapy in subclinical hypothyroidism. A double-blind placebo controlled trial. *Ann Intern Med* 1984; **101**: 18–24.

11   Arem R, Patsch W. Lipoprotein and apolipoprotein levels in subclinical hypothyroidism. *Arch Int Med* 1990; **150**: 2097–100.

12   Franklyn JA, Daykin J, Betteridge J, Hughes EA, *et al.* Thyroxine replacement therapy and circulating lipid concentrations. *Clin Endocrinol* 1993; **38**: 453–9.

13   Ross DS, Neer RM, Ridgway EC, Daniels GH. Subclinical hyperthyroidism and reduced bone density as a possible result of prolonged suppression of the pituitary-thyroid axis with L-thyroxine. *Am J Med* 1987; **82**: 1167–70.

14   Kung AWC, Pun KK. Bone mineral density in premenopausal women receiving long-term physiological doses of levothyroxine. *JAMA* 1991; **265**: 2688–91.

15   Grant DJ, McMurdo MET, Mole PA, Paterson CR, Davies RR. Suppressed TSH levels secondary to thyroxine replacement therapy are not associated with osteoporosis. *Clin Endocrinol* 1993; **39**: 529–33.

16   Franklyn JA, Betteridge J, Daykin J, Holder R, *et al.* Long-term thyroxine treatment and bone mineral density. *Lancet* 1992; **340**: 9–13.

17   Franklyn JA, Betteridge J, Holder R, Daykin J, *et al.* Bone mineral density in thyroxine treated females with or without a previous history of thyrotoxicosis. *Clin Endocrinol* 1994; **41**: 425–32.

18   Franklyn JA, Betteridge J, Holder R, Sheppard MC. Effect of estrogen replacement therapy upon bone mineral density in thyroxine treated postmenopausal women with a past history of thyrotoxicosis. *Thyroid* 1995; **5**: 359–63.

19   Cummings SR, Black DM, Nevitt MC. Bone density at various sites for prediction of hip fractures. *Lancet* 1993; **341**: 72–5.

20   Dempster DW, Lindsay R. Pathogenesis of osteoporosis. *Lancet* 1993; **341**: 797–801.

21   Surks MI, Chopra IJ, Mariash CN, Nicoloff JT, Solomon DH. American Thyroid Association guidelines for use of laboratory tests in thyroid disorders. *JAMA* 1990; **263**: 1529–32.

22   Franklyn JA, Sheppard MC. Thyroxine replacement therapy and osteoporosis. *Br Med J* 1990; **300**: 693–4.

23   Franklyn JA, Sheppard MC. The thyroid and osteoporosis. *Trends in Endocrinol Metab* 1992; **3**: 111–4.

24   Leese GP, Jung RT, Guthrie C, Waugh N, Browning MCK. Morbidity in patients on L-thyroxine: a comparison of those with normal TSH to those with a suppressed TSH. *Clin Endocrinol* 1992; **37**: 500–3.

25   Solomon BL, Wartofsky L, Burman KD. Prevalence of fractures in postmenopausal women with thyroid disease. *Thyroid* 1993; **3**: 17–23.

26   Cummings SR, Nevitt MC, Browner WS, Stone K, *et al.* Risk factors for

hip fracture in white women. *New Engl J Med* 1995; **332**: 767–73.
27 Castelli WP. Epidemiology of coronary heart disease: the Framingham study. *Am J Med* 1984; **76**: 4–12.
28 Sawin C, Geller A, Wolf PA et al. Low serum thyrotropin concentrations as a risk factor for atrial fibrillation in older persons. *New Engl J Med* 1994; **331**: 1249–52.

2 | Glucocorticoid replacement: is monitoring necessary?

James AO Ahlquist
Consultant Physician and Endocrinologist, Southend Hospital, Essex

Trevor A Howlett
Consultant Physician and Endocrinologist, Department of Diabetes & Endocrinology, Leicester Royal Infirmary

Although much has been written about the merits and difficulties involved in monitoring replacement therapy with thyroid and sex hormones, there is little consensus regarding the monitoring of glucocorticoid replacement. Yet glucocorticoids are essential to life, and there are clear and well known adverse effects from a deficiency or an excess of glucocorticoid. This chapter considers whether it is useful or necessary to monitor glucocorticoid replacement, and examines some of the evidence for the benefits of dose adjustment for individual patients.

Who needs glucocorticoid replacement therapy?

Two groups of patients need glucocorticoid replacement: patients with pituitary failure and those with primary adrenal disease.

Pituitary failure

Patients with corticotrophin (adrenocorticotrophic hormone; ACTH) deficiency, usually as part of hypopituitarism, require treatment. As a rule these patients need glucocorticoid replacement only; mineralocorticoid replacement is not required in hypopituitarism. The glucocorticoid needs of patients with established ACTH deficiency are the same, regardless of the reason for their deficiency, with one exception: patients who have had Cushing's disease successfully treated by pituitary surgery. These patients

9

often have temporary suppression of ACTH secretion and require withdrawal of replacement therapy at intervals for reassessment and so will not be considered here.

Primary adrenal disease

Patients who have had bilateral adrenalectomy, or who have Addison's disease, need both glucocorticoid and mineralocorticoid replacement. Patients with congenital adrenal hyperplasia (most commonly 21-hydroxylase deficiency) require glucocorticoid therapy both to replace cortisol deficiency and to suppress pituitary ACTH secretion: many such patients also require mineralocorticoid replacement.

Which glucocorticoid to use as replacement?

In principle any glucocorticoid drug could be used as replacement therapy. The most commonly used glucocorticoids, and their equivalent doses, are listed in Table 1. Khalid *et al.*[1] have compared the effects of these therapies in patients requiring adrenal replacement therapy. The naturally produced glucocorticoid is cortisol (perversely described as 'hydrocortisone' when formulated as a drug), and this is the glucocorticoid most commonly used for replacement therapy. It is rapidly absorbed, and so suppresses ACTH quickly and effectively,[2] but has a short half-life in plasma (90–120 minutes). Cortisone acetate, which was the original glucocorticoid used for therapy, depends on conversion into cortisol in the liver. This means that cortisone acetate has a smoother onset of action, but its bioavailability is less predictable than hydrocortisone.[3,4] Prednisolone and dexamethasone are most commonly used in higher doses for their anti-inflammatory

Table 1. Steroids used in adrenal replacement therapy

Steroids	Range of recommended replacement doses
Glucocorticoids	
Hydrocortisone (= cortisol)	15–30mg
Cortisone acetate	25–37.5mg
Prednisolone	5– 7.5mg
Dexamethasone	0.5mg
Mineralocorticoid	
Fludrocortisone	100–200µg daily

effect, but can be used for glucocorticoid replacement. They both have a more sustained inhibitory effect on ACTH secretion, and are particularly useful where ACTH suppression is important, such as in congenital adrenal hyperplasia, but dose adjustment may be more difficult and dexamethasone in particular may be associated with a higher incidence of cushingoid side-effects.

Should we monitor hydrocortisone replacement?

Once a patient is established on glucocorticoid replacement and is feeling well, is it necessary to monitor the therapy? Possible reasons for monitoring therapy are:

- Hydrocortisone is the natural glucocorticoid hormone, cortisol, and total levels of cortisol achieved in blood and urine can be measured easily by routine assays.
- Only accurate biochemical monitoring could hope to avoid minor degrees of under-replacement and over-replacement.
- There is marked variation in plasma cortisol levels between patients on an equivalent dose of hydrocortisone replacement therapy.

Clinical assessment of under-replacement

Symptoms of hypoadrenalism are typically vague: the patient might be tired, feel generally unwell, or feel dizzy, particularly on standing up, with postural hypotension; he or she might complain of headache, vague epigastric discomfort or abdominal pain. Such symptoms are non-specific, quite prevalent in the normal population and therefore cannot be used as an accurate guide to replacement therapy. The only exception might be when such symptoms were more marked just before each dose of hydrocortisone was due, and relieved after the dose.

Clinical assessment will help in severe cases of under-replacement; for example, the patient with Addison's disease who is becoming progressively more pigmented, or who has marked postural hypotension. But the most common concern is that a patient who has no marked symptoms or signs of glucocorticoid insufficiency may still be under-replaced. Apart from the general malaise that such patients may feel, it is well recognised that an acute physiological stress can lead to rapid onset of cardiovascular collapse in patients receiving insufficient glucocorticoid replacement therapy.

Clinical assessment of over-replacement

Gross cushingoid side-effects are clinically obvious, but should rarely be seen in a patient taking standard doses of hydrocortisone replacement therapy. However, it appears obvious to us that minor degrees of over-replacement that cause no physical signs might still be deleterious to the long-term health of the patient. Many effects of glucocorticoid excess alter physiological parameters that are known to affect the incidence of serious disease. In patients with hypopituitarism, hydrocortisone replacement therapy leads to a rise in systolic and diastolic blood pressure, and also to an increase in plasma glucose and insulin concentrations.[5,6] Similarly, patients with Addison's disease treated with 'standard' replacement doses of hydrocortisone have been shown to have a lower bone mineral density than the normal population; higher doses correlate with lower bone-density values.[7,8] There is a concern that over-replacement with glucocorticoids will have an adverse effect on the long-term health of the patient, even when absolute values of these measures remain within the normal range for the population. Furthermore, can we ever be sure clinically whether a mild malaise, depression, slight loss of muscle strength or tendency to overweight, all of which are very prevalent in the general population, are due to glucocorticoid over-replacement unless we measure the actual levels achieved?

How often should hydrocortisone be given?

A 'conventional' dose of hydrocortisone is twice-daily, taken as 20mg in the morning and 10mg in the evening. However, the pharmacodynamics of hydrocortisone certainly predict that, with a twice-daily regime, the morning cortisol level will be extremely high and the afternoon level very low. This has been confirmed in a controlled study of a small number of patients who had their hydrocortisone dose regime changed from twice a day to three times a day:[9] patients had better well-being, assessed by various questionnaire scales, on a three times a day regime. When initiating therapy, a starting dose of 10mg in the morning, 5mg at lunchtime and 5mg in the early evening may be recommended: the dose can be adjusted for each individual patient on the basis of clinical response and biochemical monitoring.

Monitoring hydrocortisone

Free cortisol measurements in both plasma and urine have been shown to be useful in monitoring glucocorticoid replacement therapy.[10,11] At the Leicester Royal Infirmary, hydrocortisone replacement therapy is monitored by performing a simple 'hydrocortisone day curve'. The patient performs a 24-hour urine collection for urinary free cortisol measurements the day before the profile. Collection starts and finishes immediately before the patient's morning dose of hydrocortisone. The patient then takes his or her morning hydrocortisone on rising and plasma cortisol levels are measured three times during the day: at 09.00, 12.30 (before any lunchtime dose) and 17.00 hours (before the evening dose). The patient should be euthyroid at the time of the test because of the delay in gastric emptying seen in hypothyroidism.

Interpretation of a hydrocortisone day curve

Interpretation of the day curve is necessarily a matter of clinical opinion rather than scientific fact! Criteria used are as follows:

• To avoid over-replacement: the urinary free cortisol should be in the normal range (<220nmol/day in our assay) and the 09.00 hour cortisol level should be in the normal range (250–750nmol/l in our assay) for the normal population.
• To avoid under-replacement: the 12.30 hour and 17.00 hours cortisol levels should be at least 50nmol/l (and if possible >100nmol/l).

The hydrocortisone doses and times are adjusted, if necessary, on the basis of the results of the hydrocortisone day curve, and the assessment is repeated until the optimum dose is found. The aim is to use the lowest dose that achieves satisfactory levels of hydrocortisone throughout the day. We consider that there is no need to monitor hydrocortisone levels after the correct dose has been determined, and the day curve only needs to be repeated if symptoms, signs or clinical events suggest that there has been some change in requirements.

An audit of the assessment of hydrocortisone replacement therapy

The process of monitoring hydrocortisone replacement therapy has been audited in Leicester.

A review of the notes of 37 consecutive outpatients on hydrocortisone replacement showed that 78% had at least one day curve performed. A smaller proportion (51%) had a day curve performed on their present dose of hydrocortisone. Only 11% had more than one day curve performed.

For patients on twice daily doses of hydrocortisone, the median dose was 22.5mg per day (median doses 15mg in the morning, and 7.5mg in the evening). Patients taking hydrocortisone three times per day had a median dose of 20mg per day (medians 10mg, 5mg and 5mg respectively).

Mean urinary free cortisol in both groups of patients (twice daily and three times daily hydrocortisone) was in the middle of the normal range and there was no significant difference between the groups. At 09.00 and at 12.30 hours the patients on a twice-daily regime had a slightly higher mean cortisol value, but there was no statistical difference between the groups. However, there was a highly significant difference between the groups at 17.00 hours when patients on twice-daily regimes had much lower mean cortisol levels (Table 2, Fig 1) than those on a three times daily regime.

Outcome of the day curves

How many of the patients assessed by day curves fall within the criteria given above as the biochemical goals of therapy? The urinary free cortisols are in the normal range in about 75% of patients, regardless of the frequency of dose administration. A normal cortisol level at 09.00 hours is achieved more commonly in those taking hydrocortisone three times daily than in those taking it twice a day. Comparing cortisol levels later in the day, at 12.30 hours approximately 90% have detectable plasma cortisol levels on either regime, but at 17.00 hours a clear difference appears: of those on the three times a day regime 89% have a cortisol level above 50nmol/l, compared with only 44% of those on a twice-daily regime (see Fig 2). Assessing the fulfilment of all criteria together, and using 50nmol/l as a lower acceptable limit for a plasma cortisol level, 56% of patients on thrice daily hydrocortisone were adequately replaced, and only 19% of those taking hydrocortisone twice daily.

Table 2. Comparison of mean urine and serum cortisol levels in patients in twice daily (bd) and three times daily (tds) hydrocortisone regimes

Regime	Urinary free cortisol (mmol/24h)	Serum cortisol (nmol/l)		
		09.00h	12.30h	17.00h
bd	133	546	211	69
tds	132	472	148	169
$P =$	0.48	0.15	0.05	0.001

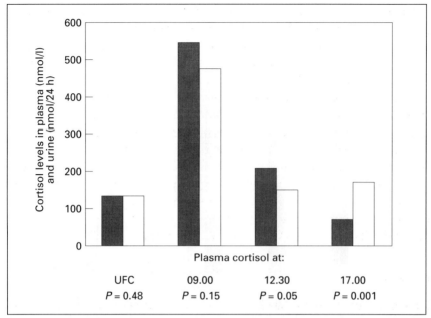

Fig 1. *Comparison of the urine (UFC) and serum cortisol levels achieved with administration of hydrocortisone twice or three times daily.* At 17.00 hours, the mean plasma cortisol achieved with twice-daily administration is significantly lower than that achieved with three doses per day.
■, twice daily; □, three times daily.

Long-term follow up

In Leicester, patients who are stable on hydrocortisone replacement therapy are reviewed annually. New action is rarely required: however, we believe that patients need to maintain contact with a specialist who can monitor routine replacement and, perhaps more importantly, can manage replacement during intercurrent illness. Hypoadrenalism is too rare for most general practitioners to obtain the necessary experience, and patients require ongoing education about adjustment of hydrocortisone replacement.

Patients should understand the importance of carrying a steroid card and/or they should have a bracelet or medallion indicating their diagnosis and replacement therapy. During intercurrent illness we normally give the following advice: for a minor illness such as a 'cold' or sore throat, there may be no need to make any change unless symptomatic; for a more severe pyrexial illness, patients should double the hydrocortisone dose for two or three days and contact the general practitioner or hospital if they fail to get better fairly quickly. Most importantly, if they have a severe

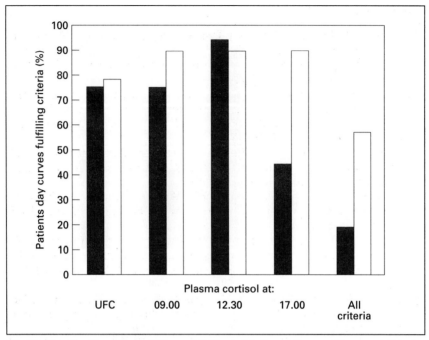

Fig 2. *Results of a review of the monitoring of hydrocortisone replacement therapy by a modified hydrocortisone day curve.* The proportion of patients fulfilling the relevant criteria (see text) are indicated. Note that fulfillment of all four criteria (with a minimum plasma cortisol level at 12.30 and 17.00 hours of 50nmol/l) was found in 19% of patients taking hydrocortisone twice daily (■), but in 56% of those taking three doses per day (□).

illness, particularly vomiting or diarrhoea, they should have parenteral hydrocortisone at home as soon as possible from the general practitioner (and/or administered by themselves or their family) and they may need to be admitted to hospital for parenteral therapy. Patients also need to know that they will need cover during surgery or for other intercurrent illness.

Conclusion

Glucocorticoid over-replacement and under-replacement may cause significant morbidity. Glucocorticoid replacement levels can be easily monitored at minimal cost. Review of the results of hydrocortisone day curves performed in Leicester supports the view that administration of hydrocortisone three times a day achieves acceptable plasma cortisol levels more often than twice daily administration. Patients on glucocorticoid replacement require long-term follow-up in an endocrine clinic.

References

1   Khalid BA, Burke CW, Hurley DM, Funder JW, Stockigt JR. Steroid replacement in Addison's disease and in subjects adrenalectomized for Cushing's disease: comparison of various glucocorticoids. *J Clin Endocrinol Metab* 1982; **55**: 551–9.

2   Feek CM, Ratcliffe JG, Seth J, Gray CE, Toft AD, Irvine WJ. Patterns of plasma cortisol and ACTH concentrations in patients with Addison's disease treated with conventional corticosteroid replacement. *Clin Endocrinol* 1981; **14**: 451–8.

3   Aanderud S, Myking OL. Plasma cortisol concentrations after oral substitution of cortisone in the fasting and non-fasting state. *Acta Medica Scandinavica* 1981; **210**: 157–61.

4   Aanderud S, Myking OL, Bassoe HH. ACTH suppression after oral administration of cortisone in Addisonian and adrenalectomized patients. *Acta Endocrinol* 1982; **100**: 588–94.

5   Matsumara K, Abe I, Fukuhara M, Fujii K, Ohya Y, Okamura K, Fujishima M. Modulation of circadian rhythm of blood pressure by cortisol in patients with hypopituitarism. *Clin Exp Hypertension* 1994; **16**: 55–66.

6   Fallo F, Fanelli G, Cipolla A, Betterle C, Boscaro M, Sonino N. 24-hour blood pressure profile in Addison's disease. *Am J Hypertension* 1994; **7**: 1105–9.

7   Yoo J, Zelissen PM, Croughs RJ, van Rijk PP, Raymakers JA. Effect of glucocorticoid replacement therapy on bone mineral density in patients with Addison's disease. *Ann Int Med* 1994; **120**: 207–10.

8   Florkowski CM, Holmes SJ, Elliot JR, Donald RA, Espiner EA. Bone mineral density is reduced in female but not male subjects with Addison's disease. *New Zealand Med J* 1994; **107**: 52–3.

9   Groves RW, Toms GC, Houghton BJ, Monson JP. Corticosteroid replacement therapy: twice or thrice daily? *J Roy Soc Med* 1988; **81;** 514-6.

10   Burch WM. Urine-free cortisol determination. A useful tool in the management of chronic hypoadrenal states. *JAMA* 1982; **247**: 2002–4.

11   Trainer PJ, McHardy KC, Harvey RD, Reid IW. Urinary free cortisol in the assessment of hydrocortisone replacement therapy. *Horm Met Res* 1993; **25**: 117–20.

3 | Growth hormone replacement therapy

Peter H Sönksen

Professor of Endocrinology, United Medical and Dental School of Guy's and St Thomas' Hospitals, St Thomas' Hospital, London

All of the chapters in this book on hormone replacement therapy are addressing issues about returning natural or synthetic hormones to people with hormone deficiencies. However, growth hormone (GH) is slightly different from the other replacement therapies described, as its use in adults is not yet widely practised: indeed, in the UK it has only recently been licensed for use in adults. Clearly it is important to consider the justification for giving growth hormone back to adults with growth hormone deficiency (GHD).

Growth hormone has been known for a long time to have major actions in stimulating long bone growth, and has been used extensively in children who are growth hormone deficient. However, its uses are now widening. It is being used in short children without GHD and also in people with Turner's syndrome, where it has been shown to increase their growth rate and almost certainly to increase their eventual height. It is also a potent anabolic hormone and is powerfully lipolytic.

The effects of growth hormone on adults are relatively newly discovered: the use of growth hormone as part of the hormone replacement regimes of adults with hypopituitarism has only recently become feasible, as a result of the unlimited amounts of the hormone that are now available through modern bioengineering. Before synthetic growth hormone was available, supplies of pituitary-derived growth hormone were so scarce that its use in children was carefully regulated and there was barely enough to meet this need.

Maurice Raben, one of the pioneers of the use of growth hormone, reported an adult with presumed GHD who appeared to obtain substantial benefit from GH administration:

'One patient, a thirty-five-year-old female, was treated in addition with GH: she noted increased vigour, ambition and sense of well-being. Observations will be needed in more cases to indicate whether the favourable effect was more than coincidental'.[1]

It has since been possible to confirm Raben's original observations through a number of well designed trials.

The syndrome of growth hormone deficiency (GHD) in adults

One study[2] has produced convincing epidemiological data that life expectancy is severely impaired in GHD. The analysis of a large cohort of GH deficient adults in and around Gothenburg, has shown that the mortality rate is twice that of the matched normal population, the premature mortality being mainly due to an excess of cardiovascular deaths, which is seen equally in men and women.[2] The definition of GHD syndrome in adults is based on the comparison of individuals with GHD and matched controls, studied in double-blind placebo-controlled trials of growth hormone replacement after full conventional replacement therapy for hypopituitarism has been given.[3,4]

In our studies, a cohort of 24 adults with severe GHD were matched with a group of healthy controls and a number of physical and psychological measurements were compared.[5] The patients had been stable for at least a year on full and appropriate hormone replacement therapy with everything except growth hormone. Growth hormone deficiency was defined as a peak growth hormone response to insulin-induced hypoglycaemia (plasma glucose of less than 2.2 mmol/l) of less than 3 mU/l.

Features of the syndrome of growth hormone deficiency in adults can be summarised:

- body composition: less muscle and more fat;
- impaired physical performance;
- reduced quality of life.

The body composition of the GH-deficient adults was abnormal: lean body mass was reduced by about 8% and their fat mass was increased by about 14% above that predicted from normal data (Fig 1). Similarly, one study[6] using mid-thigh CT scans showed that GH-deficient adults (treated with growth hormone in childhood but with no treatment for a number of years) had 63% of the cross-sectional area as muscle, compared with 85% in controls (Fig 2).

We examined muscle strength in relation to both body weight and quadriceps cross-sectional area from CT scanning, and demonstrated that patients with GHD have reduced muscle bulk

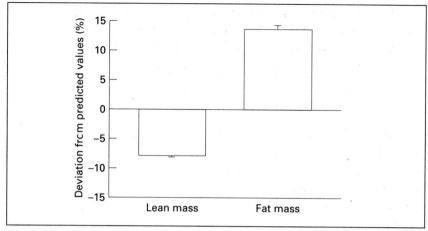

Fig 1. *The body composition of GH-deficient adults.* Adults with GHD have lower lean body mass (determined by K40 measurements) and higher fat mass than those predicted from standard reference data. From Salomon *et al.*[5]

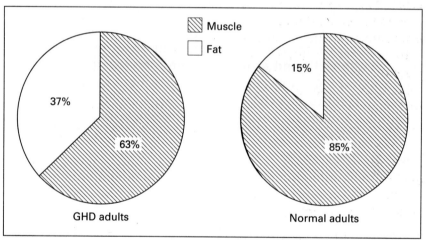

Fig 2. *Mid-thigh CT scans in GH-deficient adults.* Adults who were GHD in childhood have reduced lean body mass and increased fat mass as determined by CT scanning. From Jørgensen *et al.*[6]

and strength, and reduced force per unit area of muscle. Quadriceps force was impaired in both males and females with GHD: when corrected for reduced muscle bulk there was still significant differences in the males and nearly so in the females. We also found that the GH-deficient adults were less able to achieve predicted exercise performance, as measured by maximum oxygen uptake and maximum heart rate on bicycle ergometry (Fig 3).[7]

We also assessed 'quality of life', using three independent

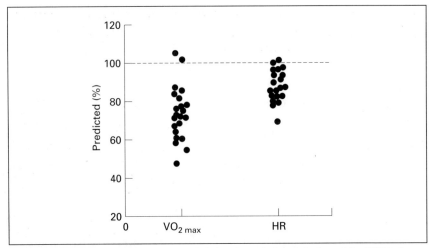

Fig 3. *Exercise preformance in GH-deficient adults.* Adults with GHD have reduced oxygen consumption ($VO_{2\,max}$) and maximum heart rate on bicycle ergometry, when compared with predicted values from control data. From Cuneo *et al.*[7]

questionnaires to measure perceived health status in our cohort of patients with GHD and in matched controls. The three questionnaires were remarkably consistent in showing a pattern of problems characteristic of GHD. Figure 4 shows one of the results taken from the Nottingham Health Profile (NHP). It illustrates one of

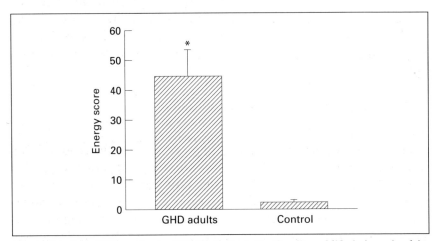

Fig 4. *Quality of life studies in GH-deficient adults.* Quality of life is impaired in adults with GHD using three independent questionnaires. The energy subscore from the Nottingham Health Profile (NHP) is higher than carefully matched controls. A high score on the NHP indicates impaired quality of life. *is significantly different from controls, $p < 0.01$.

the most consistently abnormal features found, namely an extreme lack of energy. This was one of a number of psychological features that contributes significantly to the poor perceived quality of life in GHD.[8]

Effects of growth hormone replacement in adults with GHD

Does growth hormone replacement reverse the features of GHD? The results of two independent double-blind placebo-controlled trials of six months physiological GH replacement found remarkably similar and consistent results, summarised below.[5,6]

Study design

In our study,[5] 24 patients (average age about 39 years) with adult-onset GHD of approximately 10 years' duration were randomised into two parallel groups, treated and placebo, each of six-months duration. The patients were of normal adult stature, although their body weight was about 130% of that predicted, with reduced lean body mass. They had been on replacement therapy with all other appropriate hormones for at least a year. Treatment involved a subcutaneous injection of GH (0.07U per kg per day) or placebo, given at bedtime to simulate the normal nocturnal peak of GH.

In the Danish trial,[6] patients were adults who had received GH treatment in childhood but had discontinued it on reaching final height. They differed from our patients in that, despite their GH therapy, they were still short (this has marked effects on strength, bone mineral density and work capacity). The trial was a double-blind placebo-controlled cross-over design with a 'wash out' between treatment phases.

Results of growth hormone replacement

Body composition   Within a month of starting GH therapy, mean lean body mass had increased by 5kg, with a final increase of 6kg after 6 months (Fig 5). There was a concomitant reduction in fat mass (5.5kg after 6 months), with no overall change in body weight. Figure 6 shows a mid-thigh CT scan from a representative GHD patient before, and after six months' GH replacement; the increase in muscle bulk and reduction in fat (including intramuscular fat) are easily seen. There was also a significant reduction in waist-to-hip ratio, mainly due to reduction of abdominal and visceral fat (Fig 7).[9] Growth hormone appears to be particularly effective in reducing abdominal rather than limb fat.

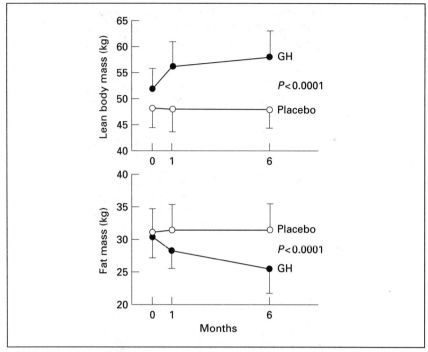

Fig 5. *The effect of GH therapy on body composition.* In a six month double-blind placebo-controlled study of GH replacement in 24 adults with GHD, growth hormone produced a rapid increase in lean body mass and a simultaneous decrease in fat mass. Body weight did not change.

Lipids Total and LDL (low-density lipoprotein) cholesterol fell by approximately 1mmol/l after growth hormone treatment (Fig 8). HDL (high-density lipoprotein) showed a gradual rise throughout the six months (although not statistically significant in this study, it has been so in others).[10]

Basal metabolic rate The basal metabolic rate rose from 1,600 to over 2,000kcal a day over the first month of GH replacement therapy. Correcting for the increase in lean body mass, the resting metabolic rate is still significantly elevated at the end of six months of GH replacement, when body composition has stabilised (Fig 9).

Exercise capacity Patients treated with GH increased their maximum oxygen uptake on bicycle ergometry to the normal value predicted for their age and body composition, with a rise in both aerobic and anaerobic thresholds.[7] Figure 10 shows the rise in power output achieved during bicycle ergometry after treatment.

Muscle strength Muscle strength was examined at 0, 3 and 6 months: there was a trend for strength to increase in all muscle

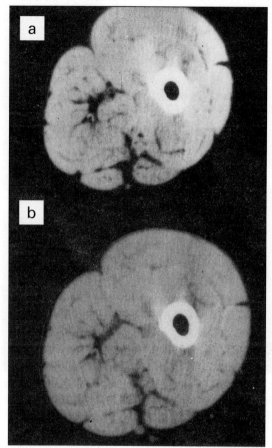

Fig 6. *The effect of GH therapy on muscle bulk and fat.* The changes in muscle and fat induced by six months treatment with GH are clearly seen on these mid-thigh CT scans; (a) untreated and (b) treated (unpublished data).

groups, with a statistically significant increase seen in hip flexion. Muscle biopsies performed at 0 and 6 months in a subset of the patients demonstrated no significant changes in muscle histology.

Cardiac changes   M-wave echocardiography revealed a significant increase in left ventricular diastolic volume, septal thickness and stroke volume at 6 months compared with baseline measurement. This is in keeping with an increase in circulating and extracellular fluid volume and an increase in cardiac as well as skeletal muscle mass.

Quality of life   Figure 11 shows the effects of GH on the energy sub score from the NHP. The high score (indicating extreme lack of energy) that was present initially in both the GH- and placebo-

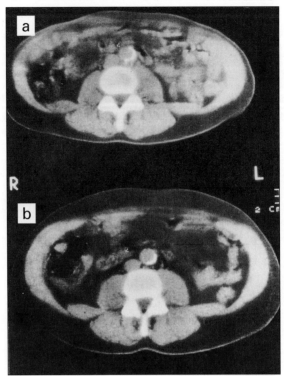

Fig 7. *The effect of GH therapy on body fat.* The remarkable changes that can occur in intra-abdominal and subcutaneous fat produced by six months GH therapy are well demonstrated in these CT scans; (a) treated, (b) untreated. From Bengtsson *et al.*[9]

treated patients returned to near zero (indicating normal perceived energy level) with physiological replacement of GH for six months. In the placebo-treated group there is a 'trial effect' of placebo injections present at one month, with no further improvement at six months. Comparable results have been reported in a large multi-centre study.[11]

Bone mineralisation Bone mineralisation was not examined in either our study[5] or that of Jørgensen *et al.*[6] However, several studies have since reported that GH replacement re-activates the bone replacement cycle in adults with GHD. Over the first months of GH replacement there is a rise in the markers of bone remodelling. Bone mineral density initially falls slightly but after six months this is followed by a progressive increase in bone density; this continues as long as GH is given,[10,12] and indeed some recent studies suggest that it continues for some time after GH replacement has been stopped.

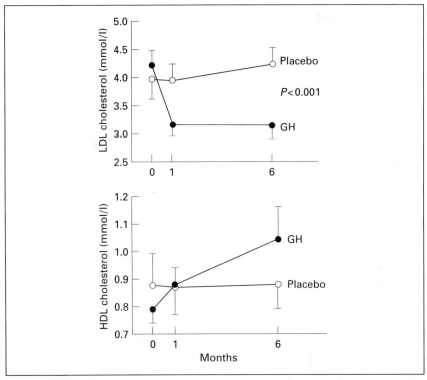

Fig 8. *The effect of GH therapy on cholesterol.* GH treatment produced a significant fall in total cholesterol, mainly due to the fall in LDL cholesterol as HDL cholesterol actually rose (not significantly in this study).

Discussion

Growth hormone is not a 'drug' but a natural substance and the results of numerous double-blind placebo-controlled trials have independently shown GH replacement in adults with hypopituitarism to have a number of significant beneficial effects. It has recently been given a product licence in the UK for use in adults. There seems little doubt to an endocrinologist that replacing missing hormones is to the long-term advantage of their patients. Now that we can be sure that growth hormone does continue to play an important role in adults, it seems only good medical practice that all GHD patients should at least be offered a therapeutic trial of GH replacement for six to twelve months. If at the end of this time, the patient and the patient's medical advisors (general practitioner and specialist) can see no tangible benefit, then it may not be worth continuing, but the possible prophylactic effect of GH replacement, against premature vascular disease and osteoporosis

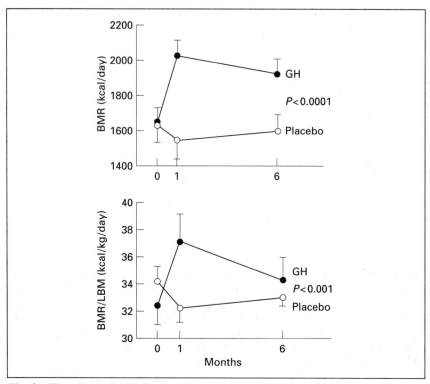

Fig 9. *The effect of GH therapy on basal metabolic rate (BMR).* Growth hormone treatment produced a marked rise in resting metabolic rate (measured by indirect calorimetry), which was sustained for six months even when corrected for the increase in lean body mass (LBM) that occurred.

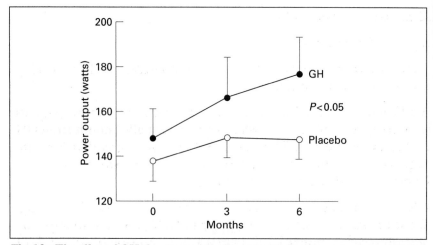

Fig 10. *The effect of GH therapy on exercise capacity.* Power output, measured with bicycle ergometry, increased on GH therapy, as did both aerobic and anaerobic thresholds.

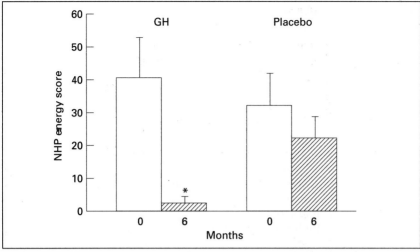

Fig 11. *The effect of GH therapy on energy levels.* An improvement in quality of life was shown in the GH-treated patients. A high-energy score indicates a lack of energy and a score of zero normal energy level. The high score in adults with GHD was normalised in the GH-treated group. There was a small but significant improvement in the placebo group ('trial effect') but this was maximal at one month while the improvement with GH continued over the entire six months of the trial.

should, however, not be overlooked. Just as with the menopause, it may not only be symptoms that justify long-term GH replacement in GHD adults.

Managing GHD in adults

A proposal for treatment

There are several steps that need to be considered when drawing up a treatment schedule.

Establish a diagnosis The first step is to identify all those patients with the syndrome of GHD who might potentially benefit from GH replacement therapy. The key symptoms and signs that indicate high risk patients are given in Table 1, with suggestions for laboratory confirmation of the diagnosis.[13]

Educate the patient The patient must be informed and educated about the significance and prognosis of GHD, and the therapeutic possibilities and potential difficulties. The possibility of a trial of GH injections should be raised.

Win the support of the patient's GP If the patient opts for a therapeutic

Table 1. The clinical features that suggest GHD in adults

History	Known pituitary pathology and/or treatment
	Full 'conventional' and appropriate hormone replacement
Symptoms	Impaired psychological well-being:
	poor general health
	impaired emotional reaction
	depressed mood
	impaired self control
	anxiety
	reduced vitality and energy
	increased social isolation
	Increased abdominal adiposity
	Reduced strength and exercise capacity
Signs	Mixed truncal and generalised obesity
	Increased waist: hip ratio
	Thin, dry skin; cool peripheries; poor venous access
	Mild or moderate reduction in muscle strength
	Moderate reduction in exercise performance
	Psychological state characterised by low, labile mood
Supplemented by test results	Stimulated GH level below 10mU/l
	Low or low-normal IGF-1
	Hyperlipidaemia (high LDL cholesterol and high triglycerides)
	Low glomerular filtration rate and renal plasma flow
	Reduced lean body mass and/or increased fat mass
	Reduced basal metabolic rate
	Reduced bone density

trial of GH replacement, we then write to the patient's GP, explaining the condition and its management and enclose a brief portfolio of key recent papers on the subject. We give details about the GH cartridges for the 'pen injectors' which, if they agree to participate, we recommend they prescribe. We offer to discuss any concerns on the phone and try to answer any questions that may arise. We ask the patient to make an appointment and visit their GP and discuss the possibility of a trial of GH therapy.

We invite the GP to play an active role in assessing the results of the treatment by using his knowledge of the patient and clinical judgement to help decide if, after a reasonable therapeutic trial, the replacement therapy with GH has been of sufficient benefit to justify long-term therapy. We often ask the GP to see the patient more frequently if there are special problems, such as hypertension, which needs to be watched closely on initiating treatment. If the GP is prepared to cooperate in the therapeutic trial, we ask them to pre-scribe an initial supply of refills for a 'pen injector'. The patient comes to the hospital to be taught how to administer therapy.

Train the patient to administer GH The patient has an appointment with a designated nurse, and brings their GH refill with them. They are taught how to make up the solution, load the pen and do the injection. This is not a trivial procedure and many patients find it quite daunting; it is much more difficult than the insulin pens. The actual injection itself is always feared but is rarely a problem. We teach the patients how to adjust the dose so that instructions for adjustments can be made by phone.

Make baseline measurements It is helpful to measure height, weight, blood pressure, body composition (impedance method under stan-dardised conditions), waist:hip ratio, plasma cholesterol and lipoprotein fractions, thyroid function tests (free T3) and insulin-like growth factor (IGF-1). In addition, full clinical photographs (with close-up of face) and completed NHP help to document the starting position and are important hard evidence to help decide whether or not there has been any benefit from the therapeutic trial. Some of the physical and mental changes that occur are remarkable and being able to refer back to baseline measures is invaluable. An up-to-date magnetic resonance imaging (MRI) scan of the pituitary is important for safety purposes and if there is any residual tumour or cyst causing or likely to cause chiasmal or optic nerve compression, full visual fields should be plotted.

Initiate GH replacement We now recommend starting at a very low dose (0.0125U per kg body weight per day, or 1U per day) and if there are no untoward effects increase the dose by 0.5U every 2–4 weeks until the IGF-1 is towards the upper end of the normal range. If the patients experience unpleasant side effects, such as oedema of feet and ankles, pains in muscles and joints of shoul-ders and hands, we ask them to reduce the dose and through grad-ual adjustment reach a dose that achieves the desired IGF-1 or the highest dose they are happy with. Much of this dose adjustment is done by discussion over the telephone, but the IGF-1 should be measured frequently and at least within two months of initiating treatment. If several dose adjustments are required in order to determine a dose that is effective and free from side effects, then more frequent IGF-1 measurements may be necessary.

Sensitivity to GH varies enormously between individuals and a patient's dose often takes a few months to become stabilised. Once this has been achieved, however, it tends to be quite stable thereafter. Patients who have previously had Cushing's disease or acromegaly seem to be very sensitive to growth hormone, often needing only a tiny dose. When small doses (0.5U per day) are needed in the long term, a 4-unit multi-dose vial and insulin syringe is more suitable than the 16U vial and a pen injector.

Monitor longer term response to GH replacement Much of the early monitoring can take place over the telephone but we schedule a hospital visit at 2 months when weight, body composition, blood pressure and IGF-1 are measured. Once therapy is stable we see the patients every three to four months and repeat these measurements and, in addition, check thyroid function tests [free T3 (fT3)]. Six and twelve months after starting GH we measure the fT3, lipids, HbA1, body composition, waist-to-hip ratio, photographs and NHP.

In addition to these measurements relating to efficacy of GH replacement, it is important to keep a watch on any remaining pituitary pathology, particularly where there is residual tumour or cyst. In these cases we repeat an MRI scan at 12 months routinely (and earlier if there is any possibility of untoward effects).

Decide if trial was effective First ask the patient if they think it has been of any benefit. In our experience, patients are extremely good observers and are usually right in their overall judgement. If the patient has close family or friends, it is worth ascertaining their views too. It is important to ask for the GP's view independently.

Objective measurements include showing:

- An increase in lean body mass, associated with a reduction of fat mass (3–5kg in 12 months is a good response).
- Change in photographic appearance, with loss of fat from face and abdomen and generally 'healthier look'.
- Reduction in waist-to-hip ratio.
- Improvement in quality of life as reflected in an improvement of mood, energy and general well-being and a fall in NHP score (this should fit with subjective assessment by patient and friends).
- Reduction in total and LDL cholesterol and rise in HDL cholesterol.

Lastly, these observations are matched with the specialist's and the GP's clinical judgement and a decision is made whether or not to continue. If there is any doubt about benefit, it is helpful to continue for another three months and review again, or to stop GH therapy and review in three months. Beneficial effects wane rapidly and several patients who, while on treatment denied GH helped them at all, changed their minds quite rapidly after it had been stopped! This can be seen in the NHP where questions exploring depression seem irrelevant when a patient is on therapy and feeling well, but can become of utmost relevance and importance within a week or two of stopping therapy if the mood deteriorates.

Long-term hormone replacement   Our earliest treated patients have been having GH replacement for more than nine years. We now have more than 100 patients on long-term replacement. For those who have been stable for several years, annual review is sufficient. The maintenance dose needed varies more than tenfold between individuals. We find that the IGF-1 values are a useful marker and quite stable over time, for a given dose. Any marked changes in the absence of an admitted dose change may indicate non-compliance. It must be born in mind that factors other than growth hormone regulate IGF-1, notably nutrition, portal insulin and thyroid status.

The dose needed for long-term replacement is not known. We have used the lowest dose that keeps the IGF-1 above the mean of the age-related normal range. This has led to good maintenance of lean body mass and quality of life but some gradual re-accumulation of fat. Whether this reflects too low a dose of GH or the normal increase with advancing years is unclear. There is some evidence from the Danish group,[6] who have maintained a slightly higher dose of GH, that they do not see the re-accumulation of fat but this may be due to their patients being younger than ours.

Dietary advice on calorie restriction should probably be part of regular counselling. Previous futile attempts at weight loss have often deterred these patients from struggling with their weight. They should be encouraged to have a further attempt since the effects of GH on the lipolytic and basal metabolic rate have produced some spectacular results! One of our patients lost more than 30kg of fat at the same time as putting on nearly 10kg of lean tissues. This had a dramatic effect on mobility and quality of life. Calorie restriction in people with normal pituitary function leads to loss of both fat and lean tissues; in adults with GHD on GH replacement you see the unique combination of loss of fat and accumulation of lean tissues.

Adverse effects   In addition to its anabolic and lipolytic effects, GH is strongly diabetogenic; as part of its action it also causes sodium retention, usually leading to fluid retention and sometimes oedema. The majority of the unwanted effects seen in early studies reflected the use of higher doses. By starting at a lower dose and increasing slowly, most adverse effects are avoided. The oedema and 'growing pains' (as several of the patients have likened them to), tend to be dose-related and self-limiting. However, they may indicate marked sensitivity requiring a dose reduction. A number of patients are hypertensive before treatment; we have not taken this as a contraindication but have managed the two conditions together with surprisingly little need for extra anti-hypertensive medication.

We have had one patient (massively obese) who developed diabetes mellitus which disappeared when the treatment was stopped. We have had a number of patients who have had headaches and recurrence of symptoms that they remember from their original pituitary problem. Most have turned out to be of no significance, but one was associated with the rapid enlargement of a residual pituitary cyst which required further surgery. It is unclear whether this was caused by the growth hormone or occurred spontaneously (as it had done in the past).

It is important to monitor thyroid function in the early stages of treatment since growth hormone stimulates the conversion of T4 to fT3 (while decreasing the formation of rT3). We have needed to reduce the thyroxine replacement dose in several patients when the fT3 exceeded the upper limit of normal. Cases of atrial fibrillation have been reported which may have been due to iatrogenic thyrotoxicosis. It seems that fT3 is the most sensitive variable to monitor. TSH is of course of no value in patients with pituitary disease.

Conclusion

The beneficial effects of growth hormone have been clearly demonstrated in many well-controlled clinical trials. Although many of these beneficial effects are tangible and well recognised by the patient, some effects, notably those affecting lipids and bone metabolism, are more subtle and only detectable with the aid of sophisticated monitoring techniques. The decision to replace GH in adults with hypopituitarism requires close cooperation between the patient, his general practitioner and endocrinologist.

Acknowledgements

I would like to thank my colleagues, particularly Dr Clara Lowy,

Dr David Russell-Jones and the research fellows with whom this work has been done and whose accumulated experience I am able to report in this paper. I would particularly like to mention Franco Salomon, Ross Cuneo, Gill McGauley and Andrew Weissberger who have worked with great enthusiasm in this new area of endocrinology and together with the rest of our endocrine team, brought us to a new level of understanding which none of us would have thought possible as recently as 1987! I would also like to thank Sue Judd, who was in 1973 our first Diabetes Nurse Specialist at St Thomas' Hospital and in 1993, as our Research Sister, became our first Endocrine Nurse Specialist!

References

1 Raben M. Medical Progress: Growth Hormone. 2. Clinical use of Human Growth Hormone. *New Engl J Med* 1962; **266**: 82–6.
2 Rosen T, Bengtsson B-A. Premature mortality due to cardiovascular disease in hypopituitarism. *Lancet* 1990; **336**: 285–8.
3 Cuneo RC, Salomon F, McGauley GA, Sönksen PH. The growth hormone deficiency syndrome in adults. *Clin Endocrinol* 1992; **37**: 387–97.
4 Rosen T, Johannsson J-O, Bengtsson BA. Consequences of growth hormone deficiency in adults and the benefits and risks of recombinant human growth hormone treatment. *Horm Res* 1995; **43**: 93–9.
5 Salomon F, Cuneo RC, Hesp R, Sönksen PH. The effects of treatment with recombinant growth hormone on body composition and metabolism in adults with growth hormone deficiency. *New Eng J Med* 1989; **321**: 1789–803.
6 Jørgensen JOL, Pedersen SA, Thuesen L, Jørgensen J, *et al.* Beneficial effects of growth hormone treatment in GH-deficient adults. *Lancet* 1989; **i**: 1221–5.
7 Cuneo RC, Salomon F, Wiles CM, Hesp R, Sönksen PH. Growth hormone treatment in growth hormone deficient adults. II. Effects on exercise performance. *J Applied Physiol* 1991; **70**: 695–700.
8 McGauley GA. Quality of life assessment before and after growth hormone treatment in adults with growth hormone deficiency. *Acta Pediatrica Scandinavica; Supplement* 1989; **356**: 70–2.
9 Bengtsson B-A, Eden S, Lonn L, Kvist H, Stokland A, *et al.* Treatment of adults with growth hormone deficiency with recombinant human growth hormone. *J Clin Endocrinol Metab* 1993; **76**: 309–17.
10 Rosen T, Johannsson G, Hallgren P, Caidahl K, Bosaeus I, Bengtsson BS. Beneficial effects of 12 months replacement therapy with recombinant human growth hormone to growth hormone-deficient adults. *Endocrinol Metab* 1994; **1**: 55–66.
11 Mardh G, Lundin K, Jonsson B, Lindeberg A (on behalf of the investigators). Growth hormone replacement therapy in adult hypopituitary patients with growth hormone deficiency: combined data from 12 European placebo-controlled clinical trials. *Endocrinol Metab* 1994; **1** Supplement A: 43–9.

12 Vandeweghe M, Taelman P, Kaufman J-M. Short- and long-term
    effects of growth hormone treatment on bone turnover and bone
    mineral content in adult growth hormone-deficient males. *Clin
    Endocrinol* 1993; **39**; 409–15.
13 Sönksen PH, Weissberger AJ, Verikiou K. Diagnosing growth hor-
    mone deficiency in adults. In: Adashi EY, Thorner MO (eds). *The
    somatotrophic axis and the reproductive process in health and disease.*
    Serono Symposia USA Norwell Massachusetts. New York: Springer-
    Verlag, 1995: 231–45.

4 | Testosterone replacement in the male: how should we monitor therapy?

Eberhard Nieschlag
Director, Institute of Reproductive Medicine,
University of Münster, Germany

Hermann M Behre
Senior Physician, Institute of Reproductive Medicine,
University of Münster, Germany

Clinical use of testosterone

The major clinical use of testosterone is replacement therapy in male hypogonadism (Table 1). All forms of male hypogonadism ranging from congenital anorchia to hypothalamic failure require long-term testosterone replacement.[1] Treatment of androgen deficiency due to gonadal failure is essential: it has well-established beneficial effects on maintenance of bone mineral density, quite apart from other effects on muscle strength and well-being. In the vast majority of patients with hypogonadism, testosterone replacement therapy is sufficient. Treatment with gonadotrophin-releasing hormone (GnRH) or gonadotrophins is appropriate only in patients with secondary hypogonadism (due to hypothalamic or pituitary failure) who require fertility. On average, this treatment phase lasts for about a year (although longer treatment may be

Table 1. Uses of testosterone in men

Clinical use	Experimental use	Disputed use	Obsolete use	Misuse
Hypogonadism	Over-tall	Senescence	Idiopathic	Athletics
Delayed puberty	stature		infertility	Body
Aplastic and	Male			builders
renal anaemia	contraception			

needed in some cases).[2] After achieving pregnancy, long-term substitution with testosterone should be continued.

Testosterone treatment in elderly men

With increasing frequency the question arises whether senescent men should be treated with testosterone replacement therapy.[3] Only few studies have addressed this question systematically.[4] While the benefits of such treatment are quite evident, there is a concern that androgen administration in older men may accelerate the age-related neoplastic changes in the prostate that are a universal feature in the elderly, leading to clinically apparent carcinoma of the prostate. This problem has not been resolved completely. Therefore, for the time being, we treat older men with testosterone only when symptoms and lack of testosterone, as reflected by low plasma testosterone levels, are present; special care has to be taken in monitoring the prostate (see below).

Other uses of testosterone

In boys with constitutionally delayed puberty short-term, low-dose therapy with testosterone may be applied to stimulate pubertal development. This is an effective treatment which, if performed properly, will not negatively influence terminal height in the boys treated.[5] Testosterone in high doses may also be given to young boys expected to develop excessively tall stature, to promote fusion of the epiphyses and thereby limit the final height attained. While this therapy results in effective reduction of final height, high-dose testosterone has no long-term side effects on testicular function.[6] In the past, testosterone was used to stimulate haemopoiesis in chronic renal failure and aplastic anaemia; erythropoietin is now widely used in these conditions, although there may be extra benefit to be derived from treatment with testosterone also. Finally, testosterone is a component of all modalities for hormonal male contraception currently undergoing clinical testing.[7] This chapter will not deal with these various uses of testosterone, nor with its abuse in athletes but will concentrate on the use in hypogonadism and the monitoring of hypogonadal patients under testosterone therapy.

Available testosterone preparations

For testosterone substitution various preparations and routes of administration can be chosen. Only the natural testosterone molecule or its esters should be used. In the United Kingdom testosterone esters for intramuscular injection, oral testosterone undecanoate and testosterone pellets for subcutaneous implantation are available (Fig 1). In addition, transdermal testosterone patches have recently been licensed and should become available in Europe soon. They are already on the market in the USA.

The most frequently prescribed forms of testosterone are the intramuscular preparations Primoteston Depot (testosterone enanthate) and Sustanon (a mixture of three esters of testosterone). The ester mixture has no clear advantage over the monopreparation. The standard dose of either is 250mg every two to four weeks.[1] For subcutaneous implants, testosterone pellets may be used (typically 600mg every four to six months).[8] Oral testosterone preparations (Restandol: capsules of testosterone undecanoate in oil) are less predictably absorbed, but are occasionally useful. To facilitate intestinal absorption into the lymph, circumventing the first-pass effect in the liver, the capsules should always be taken with a meal.[9] The transdermal testosterone system (TTS Testoderm) is applied to the scrotum and has to be renewed every day.[10,11] Of the non-scrotal patches (Androderm) two systems have to be applied simultaneously.

Further testosterone preparations are under development. Of these, intramuscular testosterone buciclate is of special interest as it produces plasma testosterone levels within the normal range for about three months and may thus reduce the injection intervals.[12]

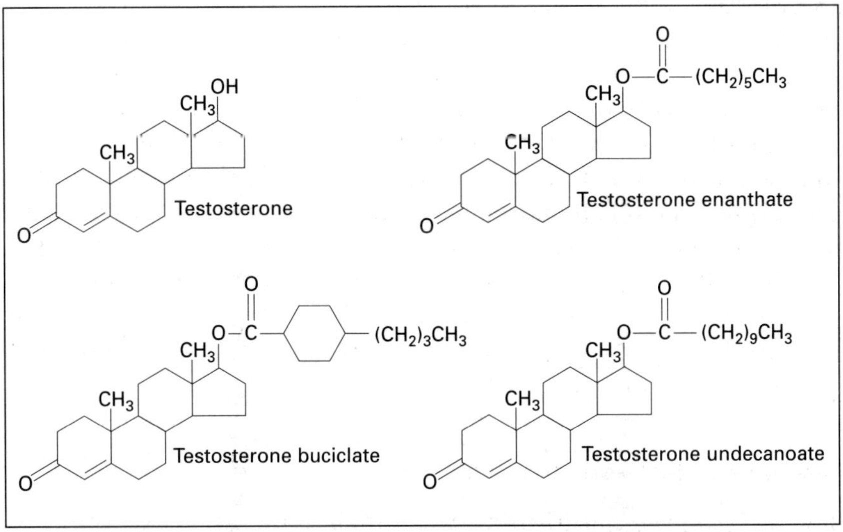

Fig 1. *Formulas of testosterone and the clinically available testosterone preparations.*

It should be noted that methyl testosterone is obsolete because of its liver toxicity. Other synthetic androgens, known mainly as anabolic steroids, have no use in the replacement therapy of male hypogonadism.

Monitoring testosterone replacement therapy

Plasma testosterone levels

Testosterone has many physiological functions[13] of which some can be used for monitoring the adequacy of replacement therapy (Table 2). However, since the therapy aims to replace the testosterone lacking endogenously, and since physiological plasma concentrations are well known, plasma testosterone levels provide a good parameter for monitoring therapy. Indeed, it was the consensus of experts attending a workshop on androgen therapy[14] 'that the major goal of therapy is to replace testosterone levels at as close to physiologic concentrations as is possible'. Following this statement, it is clear that only testosterone and testosterone esters (serving as 'pro-drugs' for testosterone) should be used in replacement therapy and that there is no place for synthetic androgens.

When plasma testosterone levels are used to judge the adequacy of testosterone substitution, it becomes clear that the available testosterone preparations all fall short of giving stable physiological levels. After intramuscular injection of 250mg of testosterone enanthate, supraphysiological plasma testosterone levels are produced for 2 to 3 days, declining thereafter to reach values below the lower limit of normal after 10 to 15 days (Fig 2).[15] Thus, depending on the injection scheme, a constant alternation

Table 2. Testosterone-dependent parameters for monitoring replacement therapy.

Physical and psychological parameters	Laboratory parameters
General well-being	Plasma testosterone,
Vigour and mood	LH (luteinizing hormone)
Body weight, muscle mass	Erythrocytes/haemoglobin/
Body proportions	haematocrit
Sexual hair pattern	Ejaculate volume
Sebum production	Prostate size
Voice	PSA (prostatic-specific antigen;
Libido and sexual activity	over 40 years)
(erections, ejaculations,	Bone density
intercourse)	

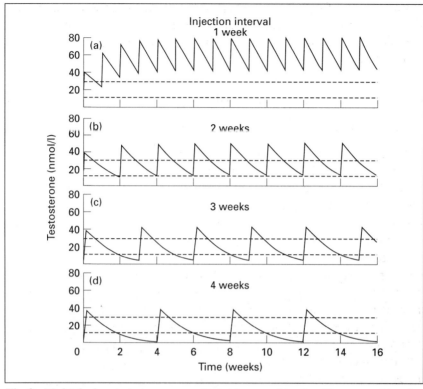

Fig 2. *Multiple dose testosterone enanthate pharmacokinetics.* Pharmacokinetics were studied after injection of 250mg testosterone enanthate (a) every week; (b) every second week; (c) every three weeks; and (d) every four weeks. ———, pharmacokinetic simulations; – – –, range of normal testosterone values. From Nieschlag *et al.*[14]

between supra- and sub-physiological levels is produced, which is closely reflected by the patients' well-being. Testosterone implants do not show the initial bursts of plasma testosterone levels, which increase at a slower rate and decline slowly thereafter.[8] Owing to the smoother kinetics, the patient experiences fewer ups and downs.

Since the pharmacokinetics for these preparations are known, and it would be impractical and uneconomic to establish a kinetic profile for each patient, it is sufficient to measure plasma testosterone levels just before the injection or implantation of the next dose. If the levels are still in the high physiological range, the dosing intervals may be extended; if the values are below the physiological range, the intervals should be shortened. This procedure can be repeated until the best scheme is found for the individual patient. This procedure may also be repeated at a later stage or when other parameters mentioned below get out of control, indicating inadequate substitution.

After oral ingestion, testosterone undecanoate produces short-lived plasma testosterone peaks which occur within one to six hours and disappear quickly; they may be in the physiological range, above or below.[9,15] For this reason, testosterone undecanoate capsules have to be given two to four times a day. Since it is difficult to base monitoring of treatment on plasma testosterone levels, other parameters are of more importance if this mode of replacement therapy is chosen. Similar short-lived testosterone peaks are produced by sublingual cyclodextrin, which have to be taken at least three times per day.[16]

Of the new preparations, the transdermal Testoderm and testosterone buciclate meet the demand of the consensus workshop quite well, since physiological plasma levels are reached.[10,11,12] Patients who received these treatments on a trial basis were very satisfied and well adjusted.

General well-being

The general well-being of a patient is a good parameter to monitor the effectiveness of replacement therapy. Under sufficient testosterone replacement therapy the patient feels physically and mentally active, vigorous, alert and in good spirits; low testosterone levels will be accompanied by lethargy, inactivity and depressed moods.[17]

Sexual functions

The presence and frequency of sexual thoughts and fantasies correlate with appropriate testosterone substitution, while loss of libido and sexual desire are a sign of subnormal testosterone values. Spontaneous erections such as those occurring during sleep will not occur if testosterone replacement is inadequate; however, erections due to visual erotic stimuli may be present even with low testosterone levels. The frequency of sexual intercourse and ejaculations correlate with plasma testosterone levels in the normal to subnormal range.[17] Therefore, detailed psychological exploration or a diary on sexual activity are useful adjuncts in assessing testosterone substitution.

These clinical experiences are substantiated by studies on androgen replacement in hypogonadal men[10,12,17,18,19] and also by recent findings in normal men in whom plasma testosterone levels are lowered by GnRH analogues.[20,21,22]

Phenotype

Muscles and physical strength grow under testosterone treatment and the patient may develop a more vigorous appearance. This anabolic effect causes body weight to increase by about 5%. Therefore, accurate recording of body weight under comparable conditions may be used as part of the clinical assessment of androgen replacement therapy. The increase in lean body mass at the expense of body fat can be measured by sophisticated techniques but this has not yet routinely been applied to the monitoring of androgen replacement.[23]

The appearance and maintenance of a male sexual hair pattern may be a good parameter for the monitoring of testosterone replacement.[24] In particular, beard growth and frequency of shaving can easily be recorded. Hair growth in the upper pubic triangle is an important indicator of sufficient androgen substitution. While women, boys and untreated hypogonadal patients have a straight frontal hairline, androgenization is accompanied by temporal recession of the hairline and, if a predisposition exists, by the development of baldness. The pattern of male sexual hair is of greater importance than the intensity of hair growth; no correlation has been found between the intensity of body hair growth and plasma testosterone levels in the normal range.[25] A well-substituted patient may have to shave daily. However, if there is no genetic disposition for dense beard growth, additional testosterone will not increase facial hair.

Sebum production correlates with circulating testosterone levels and in an early phase of treatment patients may even complain about the necessity of shampooing more frequently; they should be informed that this is a part of normal maleness. The occurrence of acne may be a sign that testosterone levels are too high: plasma testosterone levels should be checked and the dose of replacement therapy adjusted accordingly.

In sensitive patients, very high plasma testosterone levels, as may occur with testosterone enanthate, may be converted into oestrogens and thus cause gynaecomastia. This is an indication to reduce the dose or switch to another preparation. Gynaecomastia usually disappears when plasma sex steroid levels fall to normal values.

Patients who have not gone through puberty will experience voice change soon after initiation of testosterone therapy. This phenomenon is very reassuring for the patient and helps him to adjust to his environment by closing the gap between his chronological and biological age. It is specifically important for the patient to be recognized as an adult male on the phone. Once the voice has broken, it is no longer a useful parameter for monitoring the replacement since the size of the larynx, the chords and thus the voice achieved will be maintained without requiring further androgens.

Patients who have not undergone puberty before the onset of hypogonadism may also develop eunuchoidal body proportions because of retarded closure of the epiphysial lines of the extremities. Testosterone treatment will briefly stimulate growth, but will then lead to closure of the epiphyses and will arrest growth. In these patients, an X-ray of the left hand and distal end of the lower arm should be made before treatment and after the epiphysial closure further X-rays may then be taken during the course of treatment. In addition, body height and arm span, as measured from the tip of the right to tip of the left middle finger, should be measured until no further growth occurs. Continued growth, in particular of the arm span, indicates inadequate androgen substitution.

Gonadotrophins

Owing to the feedback-mechanism between hypothalamus, pituitary and testes there is a close negative correlation between plasma testosterone and both luteinizing hormone (LH) and follicle-stimulating hormone (FSH) levels in normal men. In cases with *primary* hypogonadism (i.e. intact hypothalamic and pituitary function) FSH and in particular LH increase with decreasing testosterone levels and normalise under testosterone substitution. Therefore LH may be used as an indicator of sufficient testosterone substitution. However, in cases of Klinefelter syndrome, representing the most frequent form of primary hypogonadism, LH cannot be used as an indicator of sufficient testosterone substitution since other regulatory mechanisms of pituitary function appear to be affected. Despite normal testosterone levels, LH can remain grossly elevated in Klinefelter patients (Fig 3).

Erythropoiesis

Since erythropoiesis is androgen-dependent, hypogonadal patients usually have a mild anaemia (with values in the female range) which will increase to normal values under testosterone treatment (Fig 4). Therefore, haematocrit, haemoglobin and erythrocyte count may be useful parameters for monitoring replacement therapy. If too much testosterone is administered, supraphysiological levels of haemoglobin and erythrocytes can develop, indicating that the testosterone dose should be scaled down. At the beginning of therapy we check erythrocyte values every six months, and later annually.

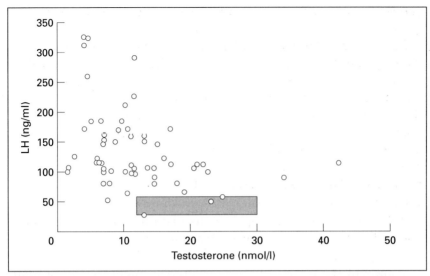

Fig 3. *Plasma LH and testosterone concentrations in patients with Klinefelter syndrome with and without testosterone replacement therapy.* The grey area indicates the normal range.

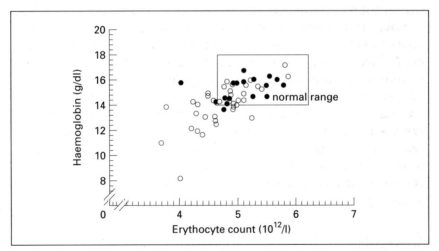

Fig 4. *Haemoglobin and erythrocytes in hypogonadal men before and under testosterone substitution.* ○, untreated patients; ●, testosterone-treated patients.

Other laboratory parameters

The testosterone preparations mentioned here have no negative effect on the liver,[26] and therefore no special monitoring of liver function is necessary. It should be pointed out, however, that 17α-alkylated testosterone preparations such as methyl testosterone are toxic for the liver and so increase liver enzymes. Their use has been discontinued (and, if not, should be) because of this liver toxicity.

Testosterone influences blood lipids and clotting factors.[22,27,28] However, these changes appear to occur within the physiological range and monitoring of these parameters is not necessary for the routine surveillance of hypogonadal patients on testosterone treatment.

Prostate and seminal vesicles

The prostate and seminal vesicles, as androgen sensitive organs, are small in hypogonadal patients and grow under testosterone therapy. Testosterone also induces their normal function as indicated by the appearance of seminal fluid. Well-substituted patients should have ejaculate volumes in the normal range (above 1–2 ml).

A study of the effects of androgen replacement on the prostate gland, by trans-rectal ultrasonography in age-matched hypogonadal and normal men, has shown that testosterone replacement does not result in prostate growth exceeding the upper normal limits; likewise, urine flow is not influenced by androgen replacement.[29] Nevertheless, rectal palpation of the prostate for size, surface and consistency should form part of the regular follow-up of patients undergoing testosterone treatment. Because of the incidence of prostate carcinoma increasing with age and the risk of stimulating such carcinoma by testosterone, patients over 40 years of age receiving testosterone treatment should be monitored at least yearly. In addition to rectal palpation we now prefer trans-rectal ultrasonography, as the entire organ can be imaged with this non-invasive technique. Serum prostate specific antigen (PSA) should also be monitored in these patients at the same time intervals.

Bone mass

Hypogonadism is associated with premature osteoporosis and increased risk of fractures. When hypogonadism is first diagnosed it is essential to assess the likely duration of androgen deficiency. If the history suggests prolonged hypogonadism, consideration should be given to assessing the degree of osteoporosis: treatment with non-hormonal methods as well as androgen replacement may be required.

Testosterone replacement in hypogonadal patients results in an increase in bone density. If this therapy is successfully undertaken before puberty, increases in both cortical and trabecular bone density occur. But if androgen replacement is delayed, mainly cortical bone density is increased.[30,31] We have measured lumbar bone density by quantitative computer tomography in over 50 hypogonadal patients before and under testosterone replacement therapy and found that adequate substitution therapy normalises bone density.[32] Since osteoporosis and the risk of fractures influence the quality of life significantly, we now subject all patients on testosterone substitution therapy to measurement of bone density every two years and take the results into consideration for the testosterone regimen. If not all patients can be monitored, we would at least strongly recommend measuring bone density in patients with long-standing untreated hypogonadism and in older patients when hypogonadism is first diagnosed. Further monitoring should then be implemented if values for bone density are subnormal at the inception of testosterone therapy.

Conclusion

Testosterone replacement is very effective in treating male hypogonadism and restores to the patient a good quality of life. Although the available testosterone preparations do not have ideal pharmacokinetic properties, patients can be treated satisfactorily if dosage is tailored to the needs of the individual patient. A wide spectrum of parameters is available to monitor replacement therapy. Once a satisfactory therapeutic regimen has been established, annual checkups at a specialised centre should be recommended, in addition to the more frequent contact with his local physician, which may occur routinely when the next dose of testosterone is administered or prescribed.

The shorter life expectancy of men compared to women is often attributed to effects of testosterone. Hence it may be asked whether testosterone may have a life-shortening effect on patients with hypogonadism under testosterone treatment. Since there are no appropriate studies available to answer this question, we investigated the life expectancy of singers born between 1581 and 1858 who were castrated pre-pubertally in order to preserve their soprano voices and compared them with non-castrated singers born during the same time. Surprisingly, there was no significant difference between the life span of intact and castrated singers, indicating that testosterone may not be a life-shortening agent.[33] Therefore, testosterone replacement therapy can be offered to hypogonadal men without hesitation, for without testosterone they would eke out a life of low quality which, to paraphrase Thomas

Hobbes (1588–1679), might be 'solitary, poor, nasty, brutish, but not necessarily short'.*

Acknowledgement

The authors would like to thank Susan Nieschlag (MA) for language editing of the manuscript.

References

1 Nieschlag E, Behre HM. Pharmacology and clinical use of testosterone. In: Nieschlag E, Behre HM (eds) *Testosterone—action, deficiency, substitution.* Heidelberg: Springer, 1990; 92–114.

2 Kliesch S, Behre HM, Nieschlag E. High efficacy of gonadotropin or pulsatile GnRH treatment in hypogonadotropic hypogonadal men. *Eur J Endocrinol* 1994; **131**; 347–54.

3 Vermeulen A. Androgens and male senescence. In: Nieschlag E, Behre HM (eds) *Testosterone—action, deficiency, substitution.* Heidelberg: Springer, 1990; 261–73.

4 Tenover JS. Effects of testosterone supplementation in the aging male. *J Clin Endocrinol Metab* 1992; **75**: 1092–8.

5 Richman RA, Kirsch LR. Testosterone treatment in adolescent boys with constitutional delay in growth and development. *N Engl J Med* 1988; **319**: 1563–7.

6 Lemcke B, Zentgraf J, Behre HM, Kliesch S, Brämswig J, Nieschlag E. Long-term effects on testicular function of high-dose testosterone treatment for excessively tall stature. *J Clin Endocrinol Metab* 1996; **81**: 296–301.

7 Nieschlag E, Behre HM, Weinbauer GF. Hormonal male contraception: a real chance? In: Nieschlag E, Habenicht UF (eds) *Spermatogenesis—fertilization–contraception. Molecular, cellular and endocrine events in male reproduction.* Heidelberg: Springer, 1992; 477–501.

8 Handelsman DJ, Conway AJ, Boylan LM. Pharmacokinetics and pharmacodynamics of testosterone pellets in man. *J Clin Endocrinol Metab* 1990; **70**: 216–22.

9 Schürmeyer Th, Wickings EJ, Freischem CW, Nieschlag E. Saliva and plasma testosterone following oral testosterone undecanoate administration in normal and hypogonadal men. *Acta Endocrinol* 1983; **102**: 456–62.

10 Bals-Pratsch M, Langer K, Place VA, Nieschlag E. Substitution therapy of hypogonadal men with transdermal testosterone over one year. *Acta Endocrinol* 1988; 118: 7–13.

11 Place VA, Atkinson L, Prather DA, Trunnell N, Yates FE. Transdermal testosterone replacement through genital skin. In: Nieschlag E, Behre HM (eds) *Testosterone—action, deficiency, substitution.* Heidelberg: Springer, 1990; 165–80.

12 Behre HM, Nieschlag E. Testosterone buciclate (20 Aet-1) in hypogonadal men: pharmacokinetics and pharmacodynamics of new long-acting androgen ester. *J Clin Endocrinol Metab* 1992; **75**, 1204–10.

---

*Leviathan, Part 1, Chapter 13.

13 Mooradian AD, Morley JE, Korenman SG. Biological actions of andro-gens. *Endocr Rev* 1987; **8**: 1–28.

14 Nieschlag E, Wang C, Handelsman DJ, Swerdloff RS, Wu FCW, Einer-Jensen N, Waites GMH. Guidelines for the use of androgens. *WHO Special Programme of Research, Development and Research Training in Human Reproduction.* WHO: Geneva, 1992.

15 Behre HM, Oberpenning F, Nieschlag E. Comparative pharmacoki-netics of androgen preparations: application of computer analysis and simulation. In: Nieschlag E, Behre HM (eds) *Testosterone—action, defi-ciency, substitution.* Heidelberg: Springer, 1990; 115–35.

16 Behrouz S, Wang C, Alexander G, Davidson T, McDonald V, German N, Dudley RE. Pharmacokinetics, bioefficacy and safety of sublingual testosterone cyclodextrin in hypogonadal men: comparison to testos-terone enanthate—a clinical research center study. *J Clin Endocrinol Metab* 1995; **80**; 3567–75.

17 Burris AS, Banks SM, Carter CS, Davidson JM, Sherins RJ. A long-term, prospective study of the physiologic and behavioural effects of hormone replacement in untreated hypogonadal men. *J Androl* 1992; **13**: 297–304.

18 Carani C, Brancroft J, Granata A, del Rio G, Marrama P. Testosterone and erectile function: nocturnal penile tumescence and rigidity, and erectile response to visual erotic stimuli in hypogonadal men. *Psy-choneuroendocrinology* 1992; **17**: 647–54.

19 Cunningham GR, Hirshkowitz M, Korenman SG, Karacan I. Testos-terone replacement therapy and sleep-related erections in hypogo-nadal. *J Clin Endocrinol Metab* 1990; **70**: 792–7.

20 Buena F, Swerdloff RS, Steiner BS, Lutchmansingh P, Peterson MA, Pandian MR, Galmarini M, Bhasin S. Sexual function does not change when plasma testosterone levels are pharmacologically varied within the normal male range. *Fertil Steril* 1993; **59**, 1118–23.

21 Bagatell CF, Heimann JR, Rivier JE, Bremner WJ. Effects of endoge-nous testosterone and estradiol on sexual behaviour in normal young men. *J Clin Endocrinol Metab* 1994; **78**: 711–6.

22 Behre HM, Böckers A, Schlingheider A, Nieschlag E. Sustained sup-pression of plasma LH, FSH and testosterone and increase of high-den-sity lipoprotein cholesterol by daily injections of the GnRH antagonist cetrorelix over 8 days in normal men. *Clin Endocrinol* 1994; **40**: 241–8.

23 Young NR, Baker HWG, Liu G, Seeman E. Body composition and muscle strength in healthy men receiving testosterone enanthate for contraception. *J Clin Endocrinol Metab* 1993; **77**: 1028–32.

24 Randall VA. Androgens and human hair growth. *Clin Endocrinol* 1994; **40**: 439–57.

25 Knussmann R, Christianssen K, Kannmacher J. Relations between sex hormone level and characters of hair and skin in healthy young men. *Am J Phys Anthropol* 1992; **88**: 59–67.

26 Gooren LJG, Poldermann KH. Safety aspects of androgen therapy. In: Nieschlag E, Behre HM (eds) *Testosterone—action, deficiency, substitu-tion.* Heidelberg: Springer, 1990; 182–97.

27 Bagatell CJ, Knopp RH, Vale WW, Rivier JE, Bremner WJ. Physiologic testosterone levels in normal men suppress high-density lipoprotein cholesterol levels. *Ann Int Med* 1992; **116**: 967–73.

28 Glueck CJ, Glueck HI, Stroop D, Speirs J, Hamer T, Tracy T. Endogenous testosterone, fibrinolysis, and coronary heart disease risk in hyperlipidemic men. *J Lab Clin Med* 1993; **122**: 412–20.

29 Behre HM, Bohmeyer J, Nieschlag E. Prostate volume in testosterone-treated and untreated hypogonadal men in comparison to age-matched normal controls. *Clin Endocrinol* 1994; **40**: 341-9.

30 Finkelstein JS, Klibanski A. Effects of androgens on bone metabolism. In: Nieschlag E, Behre HM (eds) *Testosterone—action, deficiency, substitution*. Heidelberg: Springer, 1990; 204–15.

31 Horowitz M, Wishart JM, O'Loughlin PD, Morris HA, Need AG, Nordin BEC. Osteoporosis and Klinefelter's syndrome. *Clin Endocrinol* 1992; **36**: 113–8.

32 Nieschlag E, Behre HM. Testosterone replacement therapy. In: Nieschlag E, Behre HM (eds). *Andrology: male reproductive health and dysfunction*. Heidelberg, London: Springer, 1996 (in press).

33 Nieschlag E, Nieschlag S, Behre HM. Life expectancy and testosterone. *Nature* 1993; **366**: 215.

5 | Hormone replacement therapy in the prevention of osteoporosis

Juliet E Compston
*Senior Research Associate and Honorary Consultant Physician,
Department of Medicine, University of Cambridge Clinical School,
Addenbrooke's Hospital*

Osteoporosis is characterised by reduced bone mass and disruption of bone architecture, leading to increased risk of fracture. It is now widely recognised as a major health problem in the elderly population, causing considerable morbidity and mortality and imposing an enormous financial burden on the health services. The remaining lifetime risk of fragility fracture in a 50-year-old Caucasian woman has been estimated at 17.5% for the hip and around 15% for the spine and for the radius; for fragility fracture at any site, the lifetime risk from 50 years onwards approaches 40%.[1] In the UK, approximately 60,000 hip fractures and 50,000 fractures of the radius occur annually. The corresponding number of vertebral fractures has not been accurately defined; around 40,000 are diagnosed clinically each year but this represents only a proportion of the total number since many, possibly as many as two-thirds, do not come to medical attention.[2] The total annual cost of all these fragility fractures in the UK is believed to be in excess of £750 million, the majority of which is attributable to the direct hospital costs of hip fractures.[3]

Bone mass and fracture risk

Bone mass increases during childhood and adolescence to reach a peak in the third decade of life. Following a period of consolidation, in which bone size increases by periosteal appositional growth, age-related bone loss commences, probably around the onset of the fifth decade. Overall, approximately 50% of trabecular and 35% of cortical bone in the skeleton is lost over the average lifetime of a woman.[4] During and immediately after the menopause, there is an acceleration in the rate of bone loss, with annual losses of 2–6% in the spine and 1–3% in the radius and femoral neck.[5]

The diagnosis of osteoporosis has been revolutionised by the development of non-invasive techniques which enable precise measurements of bone mass at potential fracture sites. The technique most commonly used is dual energy X-ray absorptiometry (DEXA), which can assess bone density in both the axial and appendicular skeleton.[6] Bone mass is a major determinant of bone strength and fracture risk; several prospective studies have demonstrated that a single measurement of bone mass is predictive of future fracture risk, a decrease in bone density of one standard deviation being associated with a two- to three-fold increase in fracture risk.[7–10] The strength of this relationship compares favourably with that between hypertension and stroke or lipid profile and coronary heart disease and is equivalent to an eight- to twelve-fold difference in fracture risk across the four quartiles of bone density (Table 1). Most studies indicate that the best prediction is provided by measurement at the potential fracture site[11,12] (Fig 1); the majority have been carried out in women in their 70s and 80s and more data are required to confirm if similar relationships between bone density and fracture risk are seen in perimenopausal women.

Two other risk factors for fracture have recently been identified. First, the presence of one or more prevalent vertebral fractures increases subsequent fracture risk about sevenfold, regardless of bone density; this is also true, although to a lesser extent, for non-vertebral fractures.[13,14] Second, the hip axis length is positively related to hip fracture risk, a one standard deviation increase doubling fracture risk even after adjustment for bone density and body

Table 1. The effect of a decrease in bone density on fracture risk. The results show the increase in fracture risk for each reduction in standard deviation of bone density, expressed as the odds ratio and 95% confidence interval (CI).

Reference	Site measured	Fracture type	Odds ratio (95% CI)
7	Distal radius	Non-spine	3.2 (1.2–8.2)
	Proximal radius	Non-spine	2.8 (1.0–7.6)
8	Proximal radius	Non-spine	6.7 (5.0–8.9)
9	Proximal radius	All	1.6
10	Femoral neck	Hip	2.6 (1.9–3.6)
	Lumbar spine	Hip	1.6 (1.2–2.2)
	Distal radius	Hip	1.6 (1.2–2.1)

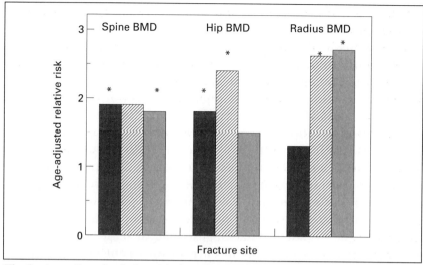

Fig 1. *Age-adjusted relative risk for spine, hip and radius fracture according to site of bone density measurement.* The figure shows the relative risk of different fractures per one standard deviation decrease in bone mineral density (BMD) according to measurement site. From data of Melton *et al.*[12] ■, Spine fracture; ▨, hip fracture; ■, radius fracture; $P<0.05$.

size.[15] This measurement, which is defined by a straight line passing from below the lateral aspect of the greater trochanter to the inner pelvic brim, can be automatically generated during routine bone densitometry.

Risk factors for falling are important determinants of hip fracture in elderly subjects. They include therapy with long-acting benzodiazepines or anticonvulsants, poor vision, neuromuscular incoordination and reduced mobility. In a recent study[16] it was shown that women with a combination of multiple risk factors and low bone density had an especially high risk of hip fracture, emphasising the importance of avoidance or treatment of these risk factors where possible.

Hormone replacement in the prevention and treatment of osteoporosis

The association between oestrogen deficiency and osteoporosis was first described by Fuller Albright in 1941[17] and has subsequently become well established. Hormone replacement therapy (HRT) prevents menopausal bone loss and reduces fracture risk at the hip, spine and radius;[18–22] however, uncertainties remain about the selection of women for treatment, the duration of treatment required for optimal protection against fracture and the non-skeletal risks and benefits of long-term therapy.

Reductions in fracture risk in women taking HRT have been shown for the hip, vertebrae and radius, mainly in observational studies. The magnitude of this protective effect is unknown; the figures of between 50 and 75% reported for hip fracture in some studies are probably an overestimate because of the confounding effects of intrinsic differences in health status between women who choose to take HRT and those who do not.[23] An important, and as yet unresolved, issue is that of the duration of therapy required to protect against fracture. At present, HRT is usually prescribed for a finite period, often between 5 and 10 years, because of concerns about an increase in the risk of breast cancer with longer-term therapy. However, some data suggest that, at least for the hip, a protective effect is seen only in current or recent users and that past use confers little protection. Given the long time period between conventional hormone use at the menopause and peak fracture incidence, particularly in the hip, it seems unlikely that five to ten years' therapy at the menopause will protect against fracture some decades later (Fig 2). A recent cross-sectional study by Felson *et al.*[24] suggests that a minimum of seven years' therapy is required for long-term preservation of bone mass; this beneficial effect was, however, limited to women aged less than 75 years at the time of bone density assessment.

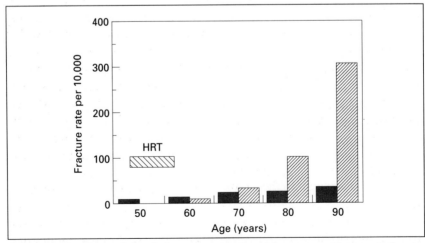

Fig 2. *Comparison of the timing of conventional hormone replacement therapy with hip and fracture incidence in women.* The figure shows the fracture incidence in postmenopausal women who had received HRT therapy. Data for fracture incidence was obtained from Kanis.[3]
■, spine; ▨ hip.

The impact of treatment with HRT depends critically on changes in the rate of bone loss following withdrawal of therapy. In a study of women who had undergone oophorectomy, bone mass eight years postoperatively was the same in women treated with oestrogen for the first four years as in those who had received no treatment, suggesting that oestrogen withdrawal was associated with accelerated bone loss.[25] Conversely, data from a cross-over, placebo-controlled study suggest that bone loss reverts to its natural rate following cessation of treatment.[26] There is a dearth of information in this area and furthur studies are required, particularly as regards changes in the spine and femur.

Strategies for the prevention of osteoporosis

The magnitude of bone loss and the severe disruption of cancellous bone structure in established osteoporosis argue strongly for a preventive approach. Criteria for the use of HRT in the prevention of osteoporosis have, however, been the subject of much debate. One possible approach is to advocate universal, life-long therapy; at present, however, this is hard to justify although it may become a serious option if the beneficial effects of oestrogens on cardiovascular and cerebrovascular disease morbidity and mortality are confirmed in prospective studies of combined therapy.[27,28] Another approach is that of population-based screening in which individuals are selected for treatment on the basis of low bone density. Osteoporosis fulfils many of the criteria required for screening; first, it has a high morbidity and mortality, second, low bone mass, which is related to fracture risk, can be assessed using non-invasive and relatively cheap techniques and third, HRT is effective in preventing bone loss and reducing fracture risk. However, the case for screening has a number of deficiencies at present.[29] Of these, the most important are lack of information about the relationship between perimenopausal bone mass and future fracture risk, uncertainty about the long-term risks and benefits of HRT and, finally, absence of established treatment protocols based on densitometric criteria.

Furthermore, because of the continuous distribution of bone density in the population and the increasing gradient of fracture risk with decreasing bone density, selection of those with the lowest bone density will have little impact on overall fracture incidence. Numerically, the largest number of fractures occur in the groups with intermediate bone density, who comprise some 60% of the population.

The potential use of bone densitometry in population-based

screening should not, however, be confused with its use in clinical practice, in which it is a valuable tool for the assessment of fracture risk in an individual. The approach currently adopted is to select women for bone densitometry on the basis of clinical and historical risk factors (Table 2). Several studies have shown that risk factor analysis has relatively poor specificity and sensitivity in detection either of low bone mass or fracture.[30-32] These findings partly reflect the varying strength and prevalence of the risk factors included in these studies, since common but relatively weak risk factors, such as cigarette smoking or a family history of osteoporosis, will have a greater influence on risk factor scores than less common but stronger risk factors such as premature menopause or corticosteroid therapy.

Clinical indications for bone densitometry

Clinical indications for bone densitometry are summarised in Table 2. For any of these, bone densitometry should only be performed when the result obtained will influence decisions about therapy; thus in most cases of premature menopause a decision to give long-term HRT can be made without recourse to bone density assessment, although the demonstration of low bone density may encourage compliance with therapy. However, for most of the indications

Table 2. Clinical indications for bone densitometry

---
1. Presence of strong risk factors
        Premature menopause (<45 years)
        Prolonged secondary amenorrhoea
        Primary hypogonadism
        Corticosteroid therapy (>7.5 mg per day for one year or more)
        Anorexia nervosa
        Malabsorption
        Primary hyperparathyroidism
        Post-transplantation
        Chronic renal failure
        Myeloma
        Hyperthyroidism
2. Radiological evidence of osteopenia and/or vertebral deformity
3. Previous fragility fracture
4. Monitoring of therapy
        HRT in patients with secondary osteoporosis
        Newer drugs, eg bisphosphonates, calcitonin, vitamin D metabolites,
            sodium fluoride
---

listed, bone densitometry is preferred to 'blind' treatment, since not all patients with these conditions will have low bone mass.[33]

Diagnostically, bone densitometry may be used to select high-risk individuals for treatment or to confirm or refute the diagnosis of osteoporosis in those with vertebral deformity, a history of fragility fracture or radiological evidence of osteopenia. In the former category, the measurement should be repeated at intervals of one to two years unless the underlying cause has been successfully treated. Bone densitometry may also be useful in monitoring the response to treatment. It is not routinely indicated in healthy peri- or post-menopausal women taking long-term HRT, although it should be performed if complicating factors are present, for example corticosteroid therapy or malabsorption. The ability of repeated measurements to indicate effects of therapy depends on the precision of the technique and the expected rate of bone loss in the absence of treatment. For example, in the spine, where precision is around 1% and menopausal rates of loss 2 to 6% per annum, effects of therapy in an individual patient can often be detected within one to two years, but in the femur, where precision is worse and bone loss in the untreated state less rapid, three or more years may be required to demonstrate significant effects of treatment.

Densitometric criteria for the diagnosis of osteopenia and osteoporosis

The gradient of increasing fracture risk with decreasing bone density is continuous and thus any cut-off level of bone density to indicate a threshold for intervention must necessarily be arbitrary. Because absolute values for bone density vary between absorptiometry systems and between skeletal sites, values are often expressed in relation to reference data as standard deviation scores. A Z score expresses the value as the number of standard deviations above or below the age-matched, mean reference value. A T score relates the bone density value to the reference range for peak bone mass in young, premenopausal adults. The use of Z scores to define osteoporosis is inappropriate since bone density decreases with age, whereas fracture risk increases; however, T scores take these age-related changes into account and are thus preferred in the definition of osteopenia and osteoporosis.

Separate thresholds have been proposed for the diagnosis of osteopenia and osteoporosis.[34,35] For the latter a T score below −2.5 is appropriate, since this will include the majority of women who will sustain a fracture and can thus be regarded as an indication for intervention (Fig 3). For the definition of osteopenia, a T score of below

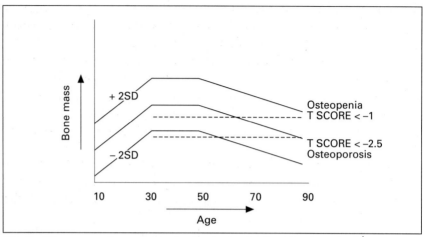

Fig 3. *Diagram to demonstrate the densitometric classification of osteopenia and osteoporosis, based on T scores.* The mean ± 2SD reference range; – – – –, show the T scores of –1 and –2.5. Data from WHO Study Group.[35]

–1, which has lower specificity but higher sensitivity, can be regarded as a reasonable criterion for prophylaxis; the indications for intervention in this category are more relative and should be influenced by other factors such as the age of the patient and the risks and benefits of the proposed treatment. It should be noted that these definitions are not applicable to men, in whom bone density values are higher.

Conclusions

Osteoporosis is a preventable disease in women, but established disease cannot be cured. Oestrogen deficiency is a major pathogenetic factor in the development of osteoporosis and HRT prevents menopausal bone loss and reduces fracture risk. Furthur studies are required to establish the optimal duration of treatment and the long-term extraskeletal risks and benefits of HRT, aspects that are likely to be interdependent; in addition, the magnitude of protection against fractures requires more accurate documentation in prospective studies.

Bone mass is an important determinant of fracture risk and the ability of a single measurement of bone mass to predict fracture has been confirmed in a number of prospective studies. Population-based screening cannot at present be justified, but this should not obscure the importance of bone densitometry in clinical practice as a means of assessing fracture risk in individual patients.

Selection for bone densitometry should be made on the basis of strong clinical or historical risk factors, in cases where the result obtained will influence decisions about therapy.

Strict densitometric criteria based on tested treatment protocols are not at present available. However, a bone density lower than 2.5 standard deviations below the mean reference value for young adults will capture almost all women who subsequently sustain a fracture and is a reasonable criterion for intervention. Prophylactic measures should be considered in women with a bone density lower than one standard deviation below the mean reference value for young adults; in such women, decisions about treatment should take into account their age and the risks and benefits of the proposed therapy.

References

1 Melton LJ, Chrischilles EA, Cooper C, Lane AW, Riggs BL. Perspective. How many women have osteoporosis? *J Bone Miner Res* 1992; **7:** 1005–10.

2 Cooper C. Epidemiology and public health impact of osteoporosis. *Clin Rheumatol* 1993; **7:** 459–77.

3 Kanis JA, Pitt F. Epidemiology of osteoporosis. *Bone* 1992; **31** (suppl 1): S7–S15.

4 Compston JE. HRT and osteoporosis. *Brit Med Bull* 1992; **48:** 309–44.

5 Dempster DW, Lindsay R. Pathogenesis of osteoporosis. *Lancet* 1993; **341:** 797–801.

6 Mazess RB, Collick B, Trempe J, Barden H, Hanson J. Performance evaluation of a dual-energy X-ray bone densitometer. *Calcif Tissue Int* 1989; **44:** 228–32.

7 Wasnich RD, Ross PD, Heilbrun LK, Vogel JM. Prediction of post-menopausal fracture risk with bone mineral measurements. *Am J Obstet Gynecol* 1985; **153:** 745–51.

8 Hui SL, Slemenda CW, Johnston CC. Age and bone mass as predictors of fracture in a prospective study. *J Clin Invest* 1988; **81:** 1804–9.

9 Gärdsell P, Johnell O, Nilsson B. Predicting fractures in women using forearm densitometry. *Calcif Tissue Int* 1989; **44:** 235–42.

10 Cummings SR, Black DM, Nevitt MC, Browner W, Cauley J, Ensrud K, *et al.* Bone density at various sites for prediction of hip fractures. *Lancet* 1993; **341:** 72–5.

11 Mazess RB, Barden H, Ettinger M, Schultz E. Bone densitometry of the radius, spine and proximal femur in osteoporosis. *J Bone Miner Res* 1988; **3:** 13–8.

12 Melton LJ, Atkinson EJ, O'Fallon WM, Wahner HW, Riggs BL. Long-term fracture prediction by bone mineral assessed at different skeletal sites. *J Bone Miner Res* 1993; **8:** 1227–33.

13 Ross PD, Davis JW, Epstein RS, Wasnich RD. Pre-existing fractures and bone mass predict vertebral fracture incidence in women. *Ann Intern Med* 1991; **114:** 919–23.

14 Wasnich RD, Davis JW, Ross PD. Spine fracture risk is predicted by non-spine fractures. *Osteoporosis Int* 1994; **4:** 1–5.

15 Faulkner KG, Cummings SR, Black D, Palermo L *et al.* Simple measurement of femoral geometry predicts hip fracture: the Study of Osteoporotic Fractures. *J Bone Miner Res* 1993; **8:** 1211–7.

16 Cummings SR, Nevitt MC, Browner WS, Stone K *et al.* Risk factors for hip fracture in white women. *N Engl J Med* 1995; **332:** 767–73.

17 Albright F, Smith PH, Richardson AM. Postmenopausal osteoporosis. *JAMA* 1941; **116:** 2465–74.

18 Lindsay R, Hart DM, Forrest C, Baird C. Prevention of spinal osteoporosis in oophorectomised women. *Lancet* 1980; **ii:** 1151–3.

19 Ettinger B, Genant HK, Cann CE. Long-term estrogen replacement therapy prevents bone loss and fractures. *Ann Intern Med* 1985; **102:** 319–24.

20 Weiss NS, Ure CL, Ballard JH, Williams AR, Daling JR. Decreased risk of fractures of the hip and lower forearm with postmenopausal use of estrogens. *N Engl J Med* 1980; **303:** 1195–8.

21 Kiel DP, Felson DT, Anderson JJ, Wilson PW *et al.* Hip fracture and the use of estrogens in postmenopausal women: the Framingham study. *N Engl J Med* 1987; **317:** 1169–74.

22 Paganini-Hill A, Ross RK, Gerkins VR, Henderson BE *et al.* Menopausal estrogen therapy and hip fractures. *Ann Intern Med* 1981; **95:** 28–31.

23 Posthuma WFM, Westendorp RGJ, Vandenbroucke JPP. Cardioprotective effect of hormone replacement therapy in postmenopausal women: is the evidence biased? *Brit Med J* 1994; **308:** 1268–9.

24 Felson DT, Zhang Y, Hannan MT, Kiel DP, *et al.* The effect of postmenopausal estrogen therapy on bone density in elderly women. *N Engl J Med* 1993; **329:** 1141–6.

25 Lindsay R, Hart DM, MacClean A, Clark AC *et al.* Bone response to termination of oestrogen treatment. *Lancet* 1978; **i:** 1325–7.

26 Christiansen C, Christensen MS, McNair PL, Hagen C *et al.* Prevention of early postmenopausal bone loss: controlled 2-year study in 315 normal females. *Eur J Clin Invest* 1980; **10:** 273–9.

27 Falkeborn M, Persson I, Adami H, Bergström R *et al.* The risk of acute myocardial infarction after oestrogen and oestrogen-progestogen replacement. *Brit J Obstet Gynaecol.* 1992; **99:** 821–8.

28 Falkeborn M, Persson I, Terent A, Adami HO *et al.* Hormone replacement therapy and the risk of stroke. Follow-up of a population based cohort in Sweden. *Arch Intern Med* 1993; **153:** 1201–9.

29 Melton LJ, Eddy DM, Johnston CC. Screening for osteoporosis. *Ann Intern Med* 1990; **112:** 516–28.

30 Compston JE. Risk factors for osteoporosis. *Clin Endocrinol* 1992; **36:** 223–4.

31 Slemenda CW, Hui SL, Longcope C, Wellman H, Johnston CC. Predictors of bone mass in perimenopausal women. *Ann Intern Med* 1990; **112:** 96–101.

32 Ribot C, Pouilles JM, Bonneu M, Tremollieres F. Assessment of the risk of postmenopausal osteoporosis using clinical factors. *Clin Endocrinol* 1992; **36:** 225–8.

33 Compston JE, Cooper C, Kanis JA. Bone densitometry in clinical practice. *Brit Med J* 1995; **310:** 1507–10.
34 Kanis JA, Melton LJ, Christiansen C, Johnston CC, Khaltaev N. The diagnosis of osteoporosis. *J Bone Miner Res* 1994; **9:** 1137–41.
35 World Health Organisation. Assessment of fracture risk and its application to screening for postmenopausal women. *World Health Organ Tech Rep Ser* 1994; No. 843.

6 | Effects of oestrogens on serum lipids and lipoproteins

David Crook
Lecturer, Wynn Division of Metabolic Medicine,
Imperial College School of Medicine at The National Heart and
Lung Institute, London

John C Stevenson
Director and Senior Lecturer, Wynn Division of Metabolic Medicine,
Imperial College School of Medicine at The National Heart and
Lung Institute, London

Post-menopausal hormone replacement therapy (HRT) with oestrogen clearly reduces the incidence of coronary heart disease (CHD) in women.[1] Oestrogen has widespread influences on various aspects of cardiovascular risk and the precise mechanisms behind this protection are the subject of considerable research interest. In addition to affecting arterial function directly (by various pathways including endothelium-dependent and calcium-dependent mechanisms), oestrogens also influence coagulation and fibrinolysis, insulin resistance and body fat distribution.[2]

The most plausible mechanism for protection involves alterations in serum lipid and lipoprotein metabolism. The initial results from the Lipid Research Clinics Program Follow-up Study[3] suggested that 50% of the protection seen in HRT users was explained by increases in serum concentrations of the potentially protective high-density lipoprotein (HDL) fraction and decreases in those of the potentially atherogenic low-density lipoproteins (LDL), although subsequent analyses have lowered this figure. Nevertheless, this is consistent with what is known of the role of these lipoproteins in the pathogenesis of cardiovascular disease.

One angiographic study[4] produced a lower estimate (25%) for the contribution of lipids and lipoproteins to the protection from CHD seen in women using HRT. However, estimates such as these arise from studies that have only made the most basic measurements of serum lipoproteins, typically LDL and HDL cholesterol alone. Recent studies have shown that oestrogen affects many other aspects of lipoprotein metabolism, such as lipoprotein(a) [Lp(a)][5] and the susceptibility of LDL to oxidation.[6] The potential contribution of these changes would not have been reflected in any analysis based on simple lipoprotein assays. Although the effects of non-lipid-mediated mechanisms are rightly of interest, the development of HRT with an optimum lipoprotein risk profile remains a priority research area.

Effects of the menopause on serum lipids and lipoproteins

The menopause induces various changes in the serum lipoprotein profile,[7,8] all of which are in a direction consistent with an increase risk of cardiovascular disease (Table 1). Increases are seen in serum concentrations of total cholesterol (mainly due to increases in LDL) and triglycerides, superimposed on the age-related increases in these lipids. Increases in Lp(a) have been reported and there may be a shift towards smaller denser LDL. Given the ability of oestrogen to increase HDL and the observation that pre-menopausal women have higher HDL levels than do age-matched men, there is surprisingly little change in HDL cholesterol concentrations during the menopause. More subtle changes, which are masked when HDL cholesterol alone is measured, may be in progress. We have described a reduction in HDL_2[8] in post-menopausal women; this subfraction may be more intimately involved in protecting against cardiovascular disease.[9]

Given the potentially adverse impact of the menopause on the serum lipoprotein profile, it seems reasonable to seek to improve this profile, especially as this can be achieved simply with therapies designed to relieve climacteric symptoms and prevent osteoporosis.

Table 1. Effects of the menopause on serum lipoproteins

Serum lipoprotein	Menopausal effects on serum levels
Triglycerides	increase
LDL	increase
Lp(a)	increase
HDL	no change
HDL subfraction 2	slight decrease
HDL subfraction 3	slight increase

Effects of oestrogen replacement therapy on serum lipids and lipoproteins

Various issues need to be addressed when considering the beneficial effects of oestrogen on serum lipoproteins. The *dose* of oestrogen is important, with larger doses tending to cause larger changes. The *type* of oestrogen may be important, with conjugated equine oestrogens having rather more effect than 17β oestradiol.[18] Above all the *route of administration* must be considered, with greater effects being seen with oral rather than transdermal or other parenteral therapies. This is due to the first-pass effect of oral oestrogen on the liver, whereby steroid concentrations in the hepatic portal vein are four to five times that in peripheral blood. The consequence of the impact of this steroid 'bolus' is to increase hepatic synthesis and secretion of a wide range of proteins.

Unopposed oestrogen therapy

HRT with oestrogen reduces serum total cholesterol concentrations by 5 to 10%, with oral therapy being somewhat more effective in this respect than parenteral therapy.[10] The higher the baseline level, the greater the fall. These changes are seen within three months of starting therapy, but their clinical significance is difficult to assess without considering the effects on individual lipoproteins and on triglycerides.

The reduced total cholesterol concentrations seen with oral therapy are predominantly due to falls in LDL. This is due to the ability of oestrogen to upregulate LDL receptors,[11] especially in the liver, and so increase the uptake of LDL from the plasma compartment. Non-oral oestradiol reduces LDL, but to a lesser extent than does oral therapy.[10] HRT affects other aspects of LDL metabolism. Oral oestrogen has been reported to reduce serum concentrations of Lp(a),[5] a particle that has been incriminated in the atherogenic process. However, this effect is often barely detectable and is not seen in all studies. The effect of transdermal HRT on Lp(a) is not known. Oestrogens protect LDL from oxidative damage,[6] a process thought to be important in the pathogenesis of CHD. Oestrogen has less effect on apolipoprotein B levels than on LDL cholesterol, due in part to a shift towards smaller, denser particles.[12] This is an unexpected finding, given that small dense LDL particles are most commonly seen in patients with myocardial infarction.[13] Recent studies indicate that the smaller particles induced by HRT are not the same as the small dense LDL seen in individuals with CHD.[14]

Oral oestrogens increase serum concentrations of HDL (especially HDL_2) both by decreasing catabolism (through inhibition of the enzyme hepatic lipase) and by increasing the hepatic synthesis of HDL apolipoprotein AI.[15] Transdermal oestrogen has less effect on HDL,[16] implying that HDL metabolism is more affected when the liver is exposed to the high doses of oestradiol.

The different forms of oestrogen used in HRT preparations differ markedly in their effects on serum triglycerides. Oral preparations of conjugated equine oestrogens (and to a lesser extent 17β-oestradiol) increase serum triglycerides due to their hepatic first-pass effect on very low-density lipoprotein (VLDL) apolipoprotein B synthesis and secretion. This presents a paradox, in that HRT reduces the incidence of CHD but women with elevated triglycerides are at increased risk of CHD,[17] especially if HDL levels are low. One explanation for this may concern the heterogeneity of triglyceride-containing lipoproteins. Kinetic studies have shown that oestrogen induces large VLDL particles which are quickly cleared by the liver and do not undergo hydrolysis to small VLDL or to intermediate-density lipoprotein (IDL), particles that are thought to be atherogenic.[18] In contrast to the effects of oral therapy, transdermal administration of oestrogen leads to a fall in triglycerides, consistent with the physiological role of oestradiol.[19]

Combined (oestrogen/progestogen) therapy

The oestrogens used in HRT increase the risk of endometrial hyperplasia and carcinoma. This can be avoided by co-administration of a progestogen. The addition of a progestogen often changes the lipoprotein profile induced by unopposed oestrogen therapy. In some cases, progestogens tend to oppose most of the effects of oestrogen on serum lipoproteins, although if the progestogen is only given for 12 to 14 days each month, as is usually the case, then this effect is only seen during the combined phase of the cycle[20] (Fig 1). It is important to note that use of a progestogen will not necessarily negate all the cardiovascular benefit seen with oestrogen, especially if the progestogen is chosen with care.[21]

Progestogens have contradictory effects on LDL. They increase the rate of formation of LDL from triglyceride-rich precursors such as VLDL, but also increase clearance of LDL.[22] Overall, these two actions appear to balance out, with the progestogens in current use for HRT and the reduced LDL concentrations, due to the oestrogen component, are maintained[23] (Fig 2). Progestogens reduce Lp(a) and therefore combinations with oestrogen will reduce

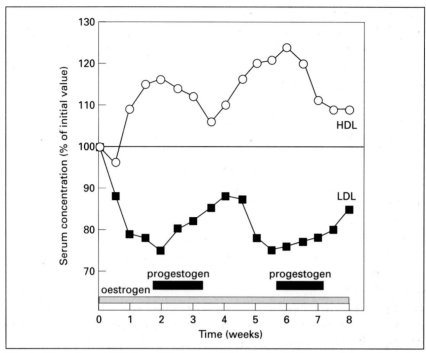

Fig 1. *The effect of HRT on HDL and LDL.* Cyclical changes in serum concentrations of HDL and LDL in women treated with oestradiol (4mg per day given continuously throughout the cycle) and sequential norethisterone acetate (1mg per day given for 10 days per cycle). Data is presented for two successive cycles of therapy. Horizontal bars indicate duration of oestrogen-only and oestrogen–progestogen phases of therapy. Adapted from Jensen *et al.*[20]

Lp(a).[7] The effects of progestogens on LDL oxidation and LDL particle size are not known.

Some of the progestogens used in combined HRT are derived from testosterone and are able to increase the activity of the enzyme hepatic lipase and so attenuate oestrogen-induced increases in HDL. Again, this is especially so in the combined phase of the cycle. In some HRT formulations the progestogen is given continuously (every day) in order to induce an atrophic endometrium. These regimens have a relatively high net dose of progestogen and so depress HDL. Avoiding the oral route by means of a transdermal system does not reduce the negative impact of norethisterone on HDL.[19] Less androgenic progestogens such as dydrogesterone, a spatial isomer of natural progesterone, do not oppose the increase in HDL induced by oral oestrogen and their use in combined HRT ensures elevated HDL levels.[24] 'Third generation' progestogens,

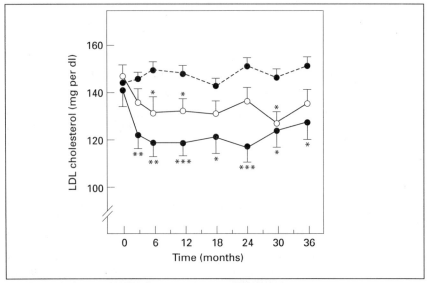

Fig 2. *Serum concentrations of LDL in women treated with hormone replacement therapy for three years.* Data are derived from the combined (oestrogen–progestogen) phase of therapy. Vertical bars represent means and standard errors. ●– –●, untreated women (*n*=29); ●—●, women treated with oral conjugated equine oestrogens plus oral levonorgestrel (n=30); o—o, women treated with transdermal oestradiol and transdermal norethisterone acetate (*n*=31). *P<0.05, **P<0.01, ***P<0.001: difference between treatment group and reference group by analysis of variance. From Whitcroft et al.[23]

such as desogestrel, are characterized by their low androgenicity and enhanced progestogenicity, despite being structurally related to testosterone, and are now being evaluated for use in HRT. Our initial experience with one of these formulations has been disappointing from a metabolic perspective.[25] Continuous combined oral oestradiol 17β and desogestrel resulted in a lowering of LDL, Lp(a) and triglycerides, but these benefits were potentially offset by marked decreases of HDL and particularly HDL_{2}.[25]

Administered on their own, progestogens tend to reduce triglycerides by reducing VLDL secretion, with the more androgenic steroids, such as levonorgestrel, being the more potent in this respect. Consequently, oral combined therapy increases triglycerides in the oestrogen phase of therapy and reduces them in the combined phase of therapy, whereas triglycerides are reduced throughout the cycle in women taking transdermal combined therapy[19] (Fig 3). HRT regimens can be tailored to provide the desired effect on lipids and lipoproteins. Thus, for a patient with elevated

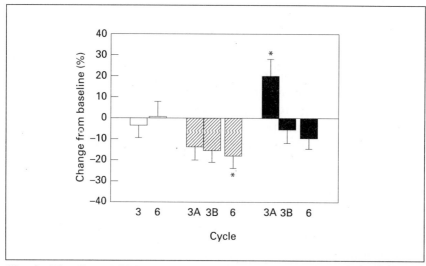

Fig. 3. *The effect of HRT preparations on serum triglycerides.* Changes (mean ± SE) in serum concentrations of triglycerides in untreated women (□; *n*=29), women treated with oral conjugated equine oestrogens plus oral levonorgestrel (■; *n*=31), and women treated with transdermal oestradiol and transdermal norethisterone acetate (▨; *n*=30). *P<0.05, significant change from baseline value compared to change seen in untreated women. During Cycle 3, subjects receiving oestrogen alone (3A), and those receiving combined therapy (3B) were studied. During Cycle 6, these women were studied whilst taking combined therapy. From Crook *et al.*[19]

triglycerides, transdermal oestradiol with an androgenic progestogen would help to reduce them, whereas for a patient with low HDL an oral oestrogen with a non-androgenic progestogen would help to increase the HDL.

Tibolone

Tibolone is a synthetic steroid increasingly used in HRT. This unusual molecule possesses oestrogenic characteristics and so is clinically efficacious in relieving postmenopausal symptoms. As this steroid also demonstrates progestogenic characteristics it induces an atrophic endometrium in many women and so does not need to be prescribed with a progestogen. Tibolone also displays androgenic characteristics in some bioassay systems. The lipoprotein profile induced by this steroid reflects these androgenic characteristics: no effect on LDL, reductions in triglycerides and HDL and substantial reductions (about 70%) in Lp(a).[26]

Conclusions

HRT affects a wide range of risk markers for coronary heart disease, as well as directly affecting the cardiovascular system itself. The ability of different HRT formulations to influence serum lipid and lipoprotein metabolism is clearly important. Careful selection of the oestrogen and progestogen components of HRT may permit optimization of the serum lipoprotein profile and ensure the maximum benefit of this therapy in terms of protection from CHD.

References

1 Stampfer MJ, Colditz GA. Estrogen replacement therapy and coronary heart disease: a quantitative assessment of the epidemiological evidence. *Prev Med* 1991; **20:** 47–63.
2 Stevenson JC. The metabolic and cardiovascular consequences of HRT. *Br J Clin Pract* 1995; **49:** 87–90.
3 Bush TL, Barrett-Connor E, Cowan LD, Criqui MH. Cardiovascular mortality and noncontraceptive use of estrogen in women: results from the Lipid Research Clinics Program Follow-up Study. *Circulation* 1987; **75:** 1102–9.
4 Gruchow HW, Anderson AJ, Barboriak JJ, Sabocinski KA *et al.* Postmenopausal use of estrogen and occlusion of coronary arteries. *Am Heart J* 1988; **115:** 954–63.
5 Farish E, Rolton HA, Barnes JF, Fletcher CD *et al.* Lipoprotein(a) and postmenopausal oestrogen. *Acta Endocrinol* 1993; **129:** 225–8.
6 Sack MN, Rader DJ, Cannon RO III. Oestrogen and inhibition of oxidation of low-density lipoproteins in postmenopausal women. *Lancet* 1994; **343:** 269–70.
7 Seed M, Crook D. Hormone replacement therapies, cardiovascular disease and plasma lipoproteins. *Curr Opinion Lipidology* 1994; **5:** 48–58.
8 Stevenson JC, Crook D, Godsland IF. Effects of age and menopause on lipid metabolism in healthy women. *Atherosclerosis* 1993; **98:** 83–90.
9 Silverman DI, Ginsburg GS, Pasternak RC. High-density lipoprotein subfractions. *Am J Med* 1993; **94:** 636–45.
10 Samsoie G. Lipid profiles in estrogen users: is there a key marker for the risk of cardiovascular disease? In: Sitruk-Ware R, Utian W (eds) *The Menopause and Hormonal Replacement Therapy—Facts and Controversies.* New York: Marcel Dekker Inc., 1991; pp. 181–200.
11 Kovanen PT, Brown MS, Goldstein JL. Increased binding of low density lipoprotein to liver membranes from rats treated with 17-ethinyl estradiol. *J Biol Chem* 1979; **254:** 11367–73.
12 van der Mooren MJ, DeGraaf J, Demacker PNM, Dehaan AFJ, Rolland R. *Metabolism* 1994; **43:** 799–802.
13 Krauss RM. The tangled web of coronary risk factors. *Am J Med* 1991; **90(2A):** 36S–41S.
14 Campos H, Sacks FM, Walsh BW, Schiff I, O'Hanesian MA, Krauss RM. Differential effects of estrogens on low density lipoprotein subclasses in healthy women. *Metabolism* 1993; **42:** 1153–8.

15 Crook D, Seed M. Endocrine control of plasma lipoprotein metabolism: effects of gonadal steroids. In: Betteridge J (ed) *Baillière's Clinical Endocrinology and Metabolism. Volume 4. Lipid and Lipoprotein Disorders.* London: Baillière Tindall, 1990; pp. 851–76.

16 Pang SC, Greendale GA, Cedars MI, Gambone JC *et al.* Long-term effects of transdermal estradiol with and without medroxyprogesterone acetate. *Fertil Steril* 1993; **59:** 76–82.

17 Bengttsson C, Bjorklund C, Lapidus L, Lissner L. Associations of serum lipid concentrations and obesity with mortality in women: 20-year follow up of participants in prospective population study in Gothenburg, Sweden. *Br Med J* 1993; **307:** 1385–8.

18 Walsh BW, Schiff I, Rosner B, Greenberg L, Ravnikar V, Sacks FM. Effects of postmenopausal estrogen replacement on the concentrations and metabolism of plasma lipoproteins. *N Engl J Med* 1991; **325:** 1196–204.

19 Crook D, Cust MP, Gangar KF, Worthington M, Hillard TC, Stevenson JC, Whitehead MI, Wynn V. Comparison of transdermal and oral estrogen/progestin hormone replacement therapy: effects on serum lipids and lipoproteins. *Am J Obstet Gynecol* 1992; **166:** 950–55.

20 Jensen J, Nilas L, Christiansen C. Cyclic changes in serum cholesterol and lipoproteins following different doses of combined postmenopausal hormone replacement therapy. *Br J Obstet Gynaecol* 1986; **93:** 613–8.

21 Crook D, Stevenson JC. Progestagens, lipid metabolism and hormone replacement therapy. *Br J Obstet Gynaecol* 1991; **98:** 749–50.

22 Wolfe BM, Huff MW. Effect of low dosage progestin-only administration upon plasma triglycerides and lipoprotein metabolism in postmenopausal women. *J Clin Invest* 1993; **92:** 456–61.

23 Whitcroft S, Crook D, Ellerington ME, Marsh M, Whitehead MI, Stevenson JC. Long-term effects of oral and transdermal hormone replacement therapies on serum lipid and lipoprotein concentrations. *Obstet Gynecol* 1994; **84:** 222–6.

24 Crook D, Godsland IF, Stevenson JC. The Cardiovascular risk profile of Hormone Replacement Therapy containing dydrogesterone: review. *Eur Menop J* 1995; **2(54):** 23–30.

25 Marsh MS, Crook D, Ellerington MC, Whitcroft SI, Whitehead MI, Stevenson JC. Effect of continuous combined estrogen replacement therapy on serum lipids and lipoproteins. *Obstet Gynecol* 1994; **83:** 19–23.

26 Rymer J, Crook D, Sidhu M, Chapman M, Stevenson JC. Effects of tibolone on serum concentrations of lipoprotein(a) in postmenopausal women. *Acta Endocrinol* 1993; **128:** 259–62.

7 | Hormone replacement therapy and cardiovascular disease: a preventive effect?

Thomas Meade
Director, MRC Epidemiology and Medical Care Unit,
Wolfson Institute of Preventive Medicine

Madge Vickers
Senior Scientist, MRC Epidemiology and Medical Care Unit,
Wolfson Institute of Preventive Medicine,
The Medical College of St Bartholomew's Hospital and the
Royal London School of Medicine and Dentistry, London

The title of this chapter suggests that there may be an element of uncertainty about the value of hormone replacement therapy (HRT) in reducing the risk of cardiovascular disease. HRT probably is cardioprotective, but the evidence for this is not as clear cut as is often assumed. It is important to keep an open mind, both over the magnitude of any benefit and also over the effects of different types of HRT. HRT began to come into widespread use in the form of oestrogen-only treatment (ORT) at a time when there was a high level of awareness of the potentially thrombo-embolic effects of the oral contraceptive preparations then in use. It was assumed that ORT might also sometimes lead to thrombotic events and consequently it was not often prescribed for or used by women at increased risk of vascular disease. This selection effect, making it likely that ORT would be mainly used by those at lower than average risk, was enhanced by a tendency for HRT users to be predominantly from upper and middle social class groups with their relatively favourable morbidity and mortality rates from a range of conditions, not just vascular disease.[1]

By the late 1970s or early 1980s, it had become clear that ORT increases the risk of cancer of the endometrium and to prevent this, many new HRT regimens included a progesterone for the last 10 or 12 days of the 'cycle'. These opposed regimens are referred to as PORT. At about the same time, reports from the early

73

case-control and cohort studies began to suggest, fairly consistently and unexpectedly, that HRT might in fact reduce rather than increase the risk of ischaemic heart disease (IHD). However, these studies were based mainly on ORT. The increasing use of PORT raised the possibility, again by analogy with work on the oral contraceptive pill, that progesterone might have adverse effects on blood lipids so that the apparently beneficial effects of ORT might be reduced or even abolished by PORT.

About 20% of post-menopausal women in their 50s and early 60s are now using HRT[2] and of course the proportion who have ever done so is even higher. By the end of the century this figure will almost certainly have risen to 30%, possibly even more. About 15% of post-menopausal women in the UK have undergone hysterectomy and about 30% of them are taking HRT predominantly as ORT. But the real, and so far largely unanswered question, concerns the 85% of women who have not had a hysterectomy and of whom about 17% are using HRT.[2] They account for more than 75% of all HRT users and their HRT is mostly in the form of PORT. It is important, particularly for a treatment involving so many people, that practice should be based on reliable information about current regimens, rather than on the potentially misleading implications of biased results from studies mainly concerned with regimens not now widely used, at any rate in the UK.

Studies of the effects of HRT on cardiovascular risk

It is frequently claimed that the cardioprotective value of HRT may be as much as 50% or even more.[3] This is almost certainly a considerable exaggeration, which has come about for a number of reasons. One is that some reviewers overlook or explain away the results of studies that do not suggest a benefit, while not applying the same standards to other studies that do seem to show benefits, although they are open to similar criticisms. Three of the cohort or prospective studies illustrate some of these issues. First is the Framingham study,[4] which initially reported an apparently adverse effect of HRT on cardiovascular risk, summarised as a relative risk in users compared with non-users of 1.9. Following criticism, an apparently beneficial effect in women under the age of 60 without angina was claimed.[5] The relative risk of cardiovascular disease in this latter group was 0.4, not statistically significant, and in older women there was an apparently adverse effect, a relative risk of 1.8, though also not significant. There is ample evidence that relying on sub-group analyses of this kind, particularly in the absence of

any prior hypothesis, is misleading. Second, interpretation of the
Walnut Creek study[6] depends on whether the analysis is based on
small numbers of events of all IHD, fatal events only or myocardial
infarction alone. Different reviews have derived relative risks ranging from 0.5 to 1.3 for different definitions of IHD.[7–10] It is clearly
important to have a common disease end-point when comparing
the results of different studies. Third, the study by Hunt *et al.*[11]
compares observed mortality in women attending special
menopause clinics with expected figures derived from mortality
rates for the whole population. While this approach may be useful
in detecting possible trends with time, the selected nature of
women not only using HRT but also attending special clinics may
lead to biased results.

It is clear from comparing the results of studies of the effect of
HRT on cardiovascular risk that the study design has a marked
effect on the relative risk recorded. The findings of various different kinds of study are given in an overview by Stampfer and
Colditz,[9] summarised in Fig 1. The six hospital-based case-control
studies indicate an increased, though non-significant, risk of
cardiovascular disease while on HRT, which was attributed to recall
bias (the tendency for patients who have had IHD to recall the use
of HRT to a greater extent than controls), and also to the difficulty
of selecting appropriate controls. In contrast, seven
population-based case-control studies, which are probably less

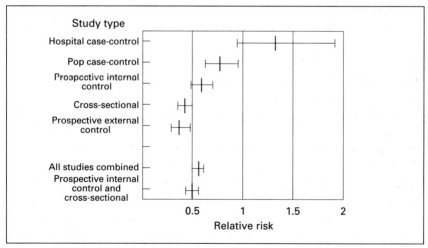

Fig 1. *Summary of the relative risk estimates and 95% confidence intervals for
studies of oestrogen use and risk of coronary disease, by study design.* There is
significant (*P*<0.001) heterogeneity of relative risks by study design.

subject to these difficulties, indicate a significant reduction in risk.

The 16 prospective studies analysed by Stampfer and Colditz (one of them[12] a very small randomised controlled trial) are divided into those with internal controls, which draw HRT users and non-users from the same population, and those without internal controls, like the study by Hunt et al.[11] already referred to, in which mortality in those taking HRT is compared with vital statistical data for the population as a whole. These latter studies (those identified as prospective external control studies in Fig 1) show the greatest apparent benefit; the prospective internal control studies also show a significant, though smaller, benefit. Finally, there are the cross-sectional studies, which use angiographic evidence of coronary artery occlusion rather than clinical disease as the outcome. These studies are not only subject to the kind of biases already referred to, they have also specifically been shown to give biased results compared with prospective studies.[13] In addition, the contribution of angiographic studies depends on views about the pathology of the final event. While changes in the vessel wall are indeed likely to be associated with an increased risk of clinical events, it is the superimposed thrombus that finally determines these, so relying on angiographic studies as a proxy for clinical events can justifiably be questioned.

In their conclusions, Stampfer and Colditz[9] considered that the prospective internal studies and the cross-sectional angiographic studies were the most reliable, giving a summary risk reduction estimate of 50%. But perhaps the most important observation in Fig 1 is the highly significant heterogeneity of the relative risks reported according to study design, which means that the results of the different kinds of studies differ significantly from each other.

Comparing study results

As there is a significant difference in results depending on the study design, which method should we rely on? Examining studies on a similar subject, the use of oral anti-coagulants after myocardial infarction, helps us to draw valid conclusions from the studies of the effect of HRT on cardiovascular risk. The analogy with HRT is really quite close. Observational studies of oral anti-coagulants include, as do the HRT studies, both case-control and cohort studies of varying quality. Moreover, in both cases several of the studies included quite extensive allowances for confounding variables, ie those associated with both the usage of the medication and with outcome (for example, low cardiovascular risk and high social class in the case of HRT and the absence of heart failure in the case of oral anticoagulants). Observational studies of the use of anticoagulants after myocardial infarction showed an apparent benefit of 50% or more. In contrast, the trials showed a reduction of 20%,[14] undoubtedly valuable but clearly much less than the benefit suggested by the observational studies. The most likely explanation for this difference is residual con founding or biases that were not (for one reason or another) allowed for. So even if the estimate of a 50% reduction in IHD associated with HRT in the observational studies can be accepted as otherwise soundly based (which, as already indicated, is questionable), it would probably be prudent to assume that the actual benefit is a good deal less.

Meade and Berra,[10] using the results of the case-control and cohort studies considered by Stampfer and Colditz[9] but not the angiographic studies or some smaller studies, suggested reductions of 25% and 20% in IHD and of 0% and 15% for stroke associated with HRT in case-control and cohort studies, respectively. Posthuma *et al.*[15] have recently compared the relative risk of all cancers with the relative risk of cardiovascular disease in all the follow-up studies of HRT included in recent meta-analyses. These imply a 35–45% reduction in the risk of cardiovascular disease in women who have ever taken oestrogens. However, in most of the studies the relative risk for all cancers was also below unity. Since the evidence is that HRT may, if anything, increase rather than reduce cancer in HRT users, these data seem to support the hypothesis of an unintended selection of healthy women for oestrogen therapy and are consistent with the suggestion that the true cardioprotective effect of ORT on cardiovascular disease has been over-estimated. So there really is considerable uncertainty about the magnitude of any cardioprotective effect, and this must be the conclusion even from the studies largely based on ORT and before considering PORT, with the possibility of adverse progestogenic effects on lipids. But with PORT there are more surprises.

Oestrogen–progesterone combination HRT and cardiovascular risk

There have been two recent prospective studies from Uppsala in Sweden suggesting potential benefit to cardiovascular risk due to PORT. They are of the prospective external-control variety, comparing observed events in HRT users (characterised by their likely self-selection and intrinsically lower risk) with regional or national rates. With this proviso, the results suggest not only that PORT may be cardioprotective[15] but that this may be due to norgestrel, an androgenic steroid considered particularly likely to have adverse effects. The same may also be true for stroke.[17] Even if selection biases partly account for the apparently protective effect of any HRT in these studies, some attention to the lower relative risks for PORT compared with ORT may be justified if these biases have affected both the PORT and ORT comparisons in the same way. Recent metabolic studies[18-20] also suggest possible advantages of PORT over ORT in the effects of the former on triglycerides and coagulability though there are, of course, many other pathways through which HRT may act.

Conclusions

It is clearly important to avoid overlooking the real possibility that HRT (again, principally ORT) may be cardioprotective. A fairly consistent finding in several studies concerned with IHD has been a gradient of declining risk from non-users to former and then current HRT users.[8,21] This certainly suggests a benefit. Overall, however, there is considerable uncertainty about the magnitude of the cardioprotective effect of HRT, particularly on the clinical question of greatest relevance, the effect of PORT in non-hysterectomised women. Medically and financially there is too much at stake for this uncertainty to be allowed to continue or for it to be resolved by unsatisfactory methods. Studies in the UK and Europe have shown the necessary randomized controlled trials to be feasible and in the US a full-scale trial is underway as part of the Women's Health Initiative. Further trials are needed and must be initiated before the general but unevaluated use of HRT in post-menopausal women makes them impossible.

References

1 Coope J. Postmenopausal oestrogen and cardioprotection. *Lancet* 1991; **337**: 1162.
2 MRC Epidemiology and Medical Care Unit. (Work in progress.)
3 Stevenson JC, Baum M. Hormone replacement therapy cardio-protective effect is genuine. *Br Med J* 1994; **309**: 191.
4 Wilson PWF, Garrison RJ, Castelli WP. Postmenopausal estrogen use, cigarette smoking, and cardiovascular morbidity in women over 50. *N Engl J Med* 1985; **313**: 1038–43.
5 Eaker ED, Catelli WP. Coronary heart disease and its risk factors among women in the Framingham Study. In: Eaker E, Wenger NK,

Clarkson TB, Tyroler HA, (eds) *Coronary Heart Disease in Women.* New York: Haymarket Doyma, 1987.

6   Pettiti DB, Perlman JA, Sidney S. Noncontraceptive estrogens and mortality: long-term follow-up of women in the Walnut Creek study. *Obstet Gynecol* 1987; **70**: 289–93.

7   Vessey M, Hunt K. The menopause, hormone replacement therapy and cardiovascular disease: epidemiological aspects. In: Studd JWW, Whitehead MI (eds) *The Menopause.* Oxford: Blackwell Scientific Publications, 1988.

8   Ross RK, Pike MC, Mack TM, Henderson BE. Oestrogen replacement therapy and cardiovascular disease. In: Drife JO, Studd JWW (eds). *HRT and Osteoporosis.* London: Springer-Verlag, 1990.

9   Stampfer MJ, Colditz GA. Estrogen replacement therapy and coronary heart disease: a quantitative assessment of the epidemiologic evidence. *Prev Med* 1991; **20**: 47–63.

10 Meade TW, Berra A. Hormone replacement therapy and cardiovascular disease. *Br Med Bull* 1992; **48**: 276–308.

11 Hunt K, Vessey M, McPherson K. Mortality in a cohort of long-term users of hormone replacement therapy: an updated analysis. *Br J Obstet Gynaecol* 1990; **97**: 1080–6.

12 Nachtigall LE, Nachtigall RH, Nachtigall RD, Beckman EM. Estrogen replacement therapy II: A prospective study in the relationship to carcinoma and cardiovascular and metabolic problems. *Obstet Gynecol* 1979; **54**: 74–9.

13 Reed D, Yano K. Predictors of arteriographically defined coronary stenosis in the Honolulu Heart Program. *Am J Epidemiol* 1991; **134**: 111–28.

14 Doll R, Peto R. Randomised controlled trials and retrospective controls. *Br Med J* 1980; **1**: 44.

15 Posthuma WFM, Westendorp RGJ, Vandenbroucke JP. Cardioprotective effect of hormone replacement therapy in postmenopausal women: is the evidence biased? *Br Med J* 1994; **308**: 1268–9.

16 Falkeborn M, Persson I, Adami HO, Bergström R *et al.* The risk of acute myocardial infarction after oestrogen and oestrogen-progestogen replacement. *Br J Obstet Gynaecol* 1992; **99**: 821–8.

17 Falkeborn M, Persson I, Terent A, Adami HO *et al.* Hormone replacement therapy and the risk of stroke. Follow-up of a population based cohort in Sweden. *Arch Intern Med* 1993; **153**: 1201–9.

18 Nabulsi AA, Folsom AR, White A, Patsch W *et al.* Association of hormone-replacement therapy with various cardiovascular risk factors in postmenopausal women. *N Engl J Med* 1993; **328**: 1069–75.

19 Caine YG, Bauer KA, Barzegar S, tenCate H *et al.* Coagulation activation following estrogen administration to postmenopausal women. *Thromb Haemost* 1992; **68**: 392–5.

20 Kroon U-B, Silfverstolpe G, Tengborn L. The effects of transdermal estradiol and oral conjugated estrogens on haemostasis variables. *Thromb Haemost* 1994; **71**: 420–3.

21 Stampfer MJ, Colditz GA, Willett WC, Manson JE *et al.* Postmenopausal estrogen therapy and cardiovascular disease. Ten-year follow-up from the nurses' health study. *N Engl J Med* 1991; **325**: 756–62.

8 | Practical aspects of hormone replacement: recent advances and the future

Margaret CP Rees
Honorary Senior Clinical Lecturer in Obstetrics and Gynaecology,
John Radcliffe Hospital, Oxford

Over the past decade there has been increasing awareness about the use of hormone replacement therapy (HRT). There are three potential benefits from the use of HRT in the menopausal woman:[1] treating the symptoms of the menopause; preventing cardiovascular disease and preventing osteoporosis.

However, the uptake of HRT is small. In Britain only 15% of women aged between 45 and 54 years take HRT (National Opinion Poll 1994) and most only take it for a few months, which denies long-term benefit, a situation that is found in many other countries. A recent survey of British women showed that the main intolerable side effect of HRT was heavy bleeding. Several studies have shown that women, have relatively little knowledge of the long-term benefits of HRT, have a variety of misbeliefs about its risks and obtain most of their information from friends or from the media. Information from a doctor or nurse, which carefully addresses the patient's needs and concerns, is more likely to result in long-term use.[2-5]

How to diagnose the menopause and when to start HRT

The age of menopause follows a normal distribution curve, with a mean of 51 years[6] (Fig 1); the age has been stable for many centuries and across ethnic boundaries. The generally agreed definition of a premature menopause is the failure of ovarian function before the age of 40, although some would use the age of 45 as a cut-off. However, the menopause can occur much earlier, even in the early 20s. Apart from natural causes of ovarian failure, there are important iatrogenic causes also, notably surgery, radiation and chemotherapy. 'Surgical menopause' applies not only to bilateral

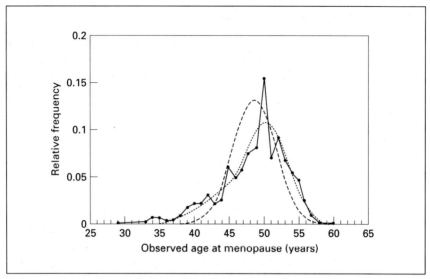

Fig 1. *The age of menopause.* Relative frequency of observed age (years) at natural menopause among Finnish women aged 45 to 64 years (*n*=907) in 1989. Shown are the original observed curve (—) and two fitted curves: (- - - -), single normal distribution; (·····), admixture of three normal curves) estimated by the C.A.MAN program. The maximum log-likelihood for the best fitting three-component solution was –2,635.762. From Luoto *et al.*[6]

oophorectomy; it is important to note that a simple hysterectomy with conservation of the ovaries advances the menopause by several years. This may go undetected because of the absence of menses as a marker of ovarian function. Radiation and chemotherapy administered in childhood also compromises ovarian function.

The best way of diagnosing the menopause is from the patient's history. Recent onset of hot flushes, vaginal dryness and infrequent menstruation in women over 40 is a classical presentation. Measurement of the serum follicle-stimulating hormone (FSH) concentration may be unhelpful since there are marked daily variations of FSH levels in the peri-menopause: values may vary from a pre-menopausal level on one day to a post-menopausal level on the next. Oestradiol levels are also unhelpful since anovulatory cycles may occur. If there is uncertainty about whether symptoms are due to the menopause, a therapeutic trial of HRT for 4 months may be the best way of establishing a diagnosis. Where premature menopause is suspected, however, it is prudent to measure a series of FSH levels because of the implications the diagnosis has for fertility.

HRT treatments: current and future

HRT consists of natural oestrogens, which must be combined with progestogens in non-hysterectomised women. Progestogens may be given either cyclically or continuously with the oestrogen. Various methods of administration of oestrogen may be used, including oral, transdermal, subcutaneous and vaginal.

Oestrogens

Several oestrogens are available for use in HRT therapy.

Natural or synthetic? Both naturally occurring and synthetic oestrogens are available for administration as drugs, but only natural oestrogens should be given as HRT. Synthetic oestrogens such as ethinyl oestradiol and mestranol are not generally used in HRT because of their greater metabolic effects. The oestrogens used include oestradiol, oestrone and oestriol: although these are naturally occurring, they are mostly produced synthetically for HRT preparations. Conjugated equine oestrogens contain a variety of oestrogens, of which the principal constituent is oestrone sulphate (50–65%).

Oral or parenteral? In choosing an HRT preparation, one of the main considerations is the route of administration. The parenteral methods give a more predictable absorption than the oral route; they also avoid the first-pass metabolism by the liver. The liver metabolises oestrogens extensively; between 30 and 90% of an oral dose may be inactivated by the liver before reaching the systemic circulation. Using oral therapy, the main circulating oestrogen is the metabolite oestrone. Furthermore, other drugs such as phenobarbitone and carbamazepine may induce liver enzymes that metabolise oestrogens, and this can reduce the efficacy of standard doses of HRT.

Oestrogens have well recognised effects on hepatic metabolism, and the use of the oral route may make these effects more marked. For example, production of coagulation factors is increased by oral oestrogen administration. No increased risk of venous thrombotic disease has been documented, but it would appear prudent to use transdermal oestrogens in women who have experienced a previous deep vein thrombosis. Similarly, high doses of conjugated equine oestrogens increase the production of renin substrate. The clinical significance is unclear, however, as the type induced is not the one normally associated with hypertension, and blood pressure does not appear to rise on this form of HRT.

Some of the effects of oestrogen on first-pass metabolism may be beneficial. The beneficial change in the plasma lipid profile is likely to contribute to the cardiovascular benefits of HRT, and it is thought that the oral route will result in greater lipid and lipoprotein changes than the parenteral routes. Both routes suppress total and low-density lipoprotein (LDL)-cholesterol, but the oral route may produce slightly more beneficial effects on high-density lipoprotein (HDL)-cholesterol.[7] Conversely, oral oestrogens increase plasma triglyceride levels while parenteral administration has either no effect or may reduce triglyceride levels. There is increasing recognition that high triglyceride levels may be an independent risk factor for ischaemic heart disease in men, though in women their role is uncertain. It would therefore be prudent to use transdermal oestrogens in women with hypertriglyceridaemia.

There has been much debate about the relative merits of oral, transdermal and subcutaneous administration of oestrogens. However, it should be remembered that the long-term benefits and safety of oral oestrogen are well-established. Furthermore, all oestrogens eventually pass through the liver and are recycled by the entero-hepatic circulation, regardless of the route of administration.

It should also be remembered that there is a wide variation in absorption and metabolism of oestrogens with any preparation and route. Thus a wide range in values is achieved. A wide range of plasma levels of oestradiol may be achieved by both the transdermal patch and oral therapy; in general, however, the plasma levels are similar to those in the follicular phase of the menstrual cycle.

Oral oestrogens The principal oral oestrogens used in HRT are oestradiol valerate, micronised oestradiol and conjugated equine oestrogens. The daily dose required to prevent bone loss is 2mg of oestradiol or 0.625mg of conjugated equine oestrogens.[1]

Transdermal oestradiol patch and gel Oestradiol is lipid soluble and can penetrate through the skin only if dissolved in an appropriate transport medium such as ethanol. Until recently, transdermal patches were only available with oestradiol contained in an alcohol-based reservoir with an adhesive outer ring. A problem with these patches is that they tend to fall off, and can cause skin reactions (with rates of up to 30% being reported). However, new technology has resulted in the development of several types of oestradiol matrix patches, in which the oestrogen is evenly distributed throughout the adhesive matrix. The adhesive properties of the matrix patch are much greater, and skin reaction are also reduced (to 5% or less).[8] A constant dose of oestradiol is delivered and patches are changed either once or twice weekly. The dose required to prevent bone loss is achieved by delivering 50µg of oestradiol into the circulation over a 24-hour period.

Oestradiol is also available in a transdermal gel which is rubbed on the skin on a daily basis. Allergic reactions are extremely rare. Both patches and gel are useful options to consider in women who have had problems with tachyphylaxis when using oestradiol implants (see below).

Oestradiol implants Oestradiol implants are crystalline pellets of oestradiol which are inserted subcutaneously under local anaesthetic and slowly release oestradiol over many months. Three doses are available (25mg, 50mg and 100mg), the higher doses giving a longer duration of action. Implants have the advantage that, once inserted, the patient does not have to remember to take medication. However, there are concerns that implants may remain effective for a very long time. It has been reported that oestrogenic activity sufficient to cause endometrial stimulation may continue for up to 3 years after the last insertion, a factor that should be taken into account in non-hysterectomised women.

Another concern with implants is tachyphylaxis: the recurrence of menopausal symptoms while the implant is still producing adequate levels of oestradiol. This results in women asking for repeat implants with increasing frequency, and a progressive increase in oestradiol levels, which eventually reach supra-physiological ranges.[9] The effect of these high levels is unknown. Tachyphylaxis can be avoided with appropriate pre-treatment counselling and, where necessary, more monitoring of oestradiol levels in women receiving implants. This is especially important in those coming back less than 6 months after the last implant.

Vaginal oestrogen Some women complain only of vaginal symptoms. These women are often many years post-menopausal and do not wish to take systemic HRT (not least because of the return of menses). For such patients a local vaginal oestrogen (in cream, pessary, tablet or ring form) is all that is necessary. As with systemic administration, it is important to give only natural and not synthetic oestrogens, since systemic absorption can occur, with potential effects on the endometrium. Oestriol can be given in a cream or pessary. It is such a weak oestrogen that it may be used (in specialised clinics) for women who have had a previous breast carcinoma. Low-dose oestradiol may be given either as a vaginal tablet; or as a vaginal ring which is changed every 3 months.

Progestogens

Several progestogens are available for use in HRT preparations.

Types of progestogen The progestogens used in HRT are synthetic. They are mainly taken in tablet form at present, though norethisterone is also available in an alcohol-reservoir transdermal patch, combined with oestradiol. Pure progesterone formulated as a pessary may be used vaginally or rectally, but currently it is not widely used in HRT. The progestogen levonorgestrel can also be delivered by an intrauterine contraceptive device.[10]

Progestogens are of two main kinds: 17-hydroxyprogesterone derivatives (dydrogesterone, medroxy-progesterone acetate) and 19-nortestosterone derivatives (norethisterone, norgestrel).

The 17-hydroxyprogesterone derivatives are not significantly androgenic, and should have no adverse effect on blood lipids. The 19-nortestosterone derivatives are more androgenic, and could potentially have an adverse effect by reducing HDL-cholesterol when combined with oestrogen. However, metabolic studies suggest that if the daily progestogen dose is reduced to 0.15mg norgestrel or 1mg norethisterone, the effect on lipids is minimal. The new generation of progestogens such as gestodene, desogestrel and norgestimate, used in oral contraceptives, are not currently available in HRT.

Oestrogen and progestogen—combinations

Progestogens are added to oestrogens to prevent the increased risk of endometrial hyperplasia and carcinoma which occurs with unopposed oestrogen and need not be given to women who have undergone hysterectomy.[11,12] Progestogen can be given for 10–12 days every 4 weeks, or for 14 days every 13 weeks or every day continuously. The first leads to monthly bleeds, the second to 3-monthly bleeds and the last aims to achieve amenorrhoea.[13–17] In the past year, the number of prepacked HRTs has increased which will hopefully help in prescribing. The return of menstruation is one of the unwelcome consequences of sequential combined HRT, and the possibility of an amenorrhoeic regimen is always welcome. Amenorrhoea may be achieved if oestrogen and progestogen are administered continuously. A typical dose for continuous administration of progestogen is 1mg of norethisterone or 5mg of medroxyprogesterone acetate daily.[15,17–19] However, amenorrhoea regimes do not suit all women: some bleed erratically and profusely for reasons that are unclear. Amenorrhoea regimes are particularly unsuitable in the peri-menopausal phase since here the incidence of irregular bleeding is high: they are only suitable for established post-menopausal women. Some may wish to start with a cyclic regime in the peri-menopause and later switch to a continuous regime.

The use of a levonorgestrel contraceptive delivery system will lead to amenorrhoea and can be used in peri-menopausal women. Here it will also address the problem of contraception.

Other HRT treatments

Tibolone

Tibolone has mixed oestrogenic, progestogenic and androgenic actions and is used in women who wish to have amenorrhoea.[20] It is administered continuously (2.5mg daily). It is used to treat vaso-motor, psychological and libido problems. It may also be helpful for the prevention of osteoporosis since studies suggest it reduces bone loss.[21] As with other amenorrhoeic regimes, use in the peri-menopausal phase can lead to irregular and troublesome vaginal bleeding; it is best used in post-menopausal women with 1 year or more of amenorrhoea.

Testosterone

The role of testosterone in women is uncertain, but it may be involved in libido and energy levels. Testosterone production falls at the menopause. Testosterone used in HRT is administered as an implant, 100mg being given every 6–12 months. It may be used in women in whom lack of libido or low energy levels do not respond to oestrogen. Plasma testosterone levels can become elevated above the normal pre-menopausal range, but complaints of androgenic side effects are rare.

Previous endometrial resection

Women who have undergone endometrial resection or ablation may wonder if they can be regarded as having had a hysterectomy, and so avoid the need for progestogen administration. However, it is not safe to assume that all the endometrium will have been removed even in women who have been rendered amenorrhoeic by this procedure. It is therefore advisable to oppose the oestrogens with progestogen.

Conclusion

There have been a number of recent advances in the methods of delivery used in HRT, and the combinations of oestrogen and progestogen. Counselling is essential to find an appropriate HRT for an individual woman, otherwise it is unlikely she will use it for an effective duration. Women often stop therapy after a few months; furthermore, only 49% of women find that their most useful sources of information are health care professionals.[5] It is essential that the endpoints of symptom control and cardiovascular and skeletal protection as opposed to the small increased risk of breast cancer be discussed. Several options are in development: use of third generation gestagens, gestagens in matrix patches, and silastic implants to deliver oestradiol.[22] While these developments will increase treatment modalities, the key role of individual discussion in advising treatment cannot be underestimated, otherwise they will not be used.

References and further reading

1   Belchetz P. Hormonal treatment of postmenopausal women. *New Eng J Med* 1994; **330**: 1062–71.
2   Barlow DH, Brockie JA, Rees MCP. Study of general practice consultations and menopausal problems. *Br Med J* 1991; **302**: 274–6.
3   Kadri AZ. Hormone replacement therapy—a survey of perimenopausal women in a community setting. *Br J Gen Practice* 1991; **41**: 109–12.
4   Coope J, Marsh J. Can we improve compliance with long-term HRT? *Maturitas* 1992; **15**: 151–8.
5   Hope S, Rees M. Why do British women start and stop hormone replacement therapy? *J Brit Menopause Soc* 1995; **1**: 26–7.
6   Luoto R, Kaprio J, Uutela A. Age at natural menopause and sociodemographic status in Finland. *Am J Epidemiol* 1994; **139**: 64–76.
7   Crook D, Cust MP, Gangar KF, Worthington M *et al.* Comparison of transdermal and oral estrogen-progestin replacement therapy: effects on serum lipids and lipoproteins. *Am J Obstet Gynecol* 1992; **166**: 950–5.
8   Pornel B, Genazzani AR, Costes D, Dain MP *et al.* Efficacy and tolerability of Menorest® 50 compared with estraderm® TTS 50 in the treatment of postmenopausal symptoms. A randomised multicenter parallel group study. *Maturitas* 1995; **22**: 207–18.
9   Gangar K, Cust M, Whitehead MI. Symptoms of oestrogen deficiency associated with supraphysiological plasma oestradiol concentrations in women with oestradiol implants. *BMJ* 1989; **299**: 601–2.
10 Andersson K, Mattson LA, Rybo G, Stadberg E (1992). Intrauterine release of levonorgestrel—a new way of adding progestogen in hormone replacement therapy. *Obstet Gynecol* 1992; **79**: 963–7.
11 The writing group for the PEPI trial. Effects of estrogen or estrogen/progestin regimens on heart disease risk factors in postmenopausal women *JAMA* 1995; **273**: 199–208.

12 Grady D, Gebretsadik T, Kerlikowske K, Ernster V, Petitti D. Hormone replacement therapy and endometrial cancer risk: a meta-analysis. *Obstet Gynecol* 1995; **85**: 304–13.
13 Rees MCP, Barlow DH. Quantition of hormone replacement induced withdrawal bleeds. *Br J Obstet Gynaecol* 1991; **98**: 106–7.
14 Rees MCP. On menstrual bleeding with hormone replacement therapy. *Lancet* 1994; **343**: 250.
15 Woodruff JD, Pickar JH. Incidence of endometrial hyperplasia in postmenopausal women taking conjugated oestrogens (Premarin) with medroxyprogesterone acetate or conjugated oestrogens alone. *Am J Obstet Gynecol* 1994; **170**: 1213–23.
16 Hirvonen E, Salmi T, Puolakka J, Heikkinen J, Granfors E, *et al.* Can progestin be limited to every third month only in postmenopausal women taking oestrogen? *Maturitas* 1995; **21**: 39–44.
17 Udoff L, Langenberg P, Adashi Ey. Combined continuous hormone replacement therapy: a critical review. *Obstet Gynecol* 1995; **86**: 306–16.
18 Christiansen C, Riis BJ. Five years with continuous combined oestrogen/progestogen therapy. Effects on calcium metabolism, lipoproteins, and bleeding pattern. *Br J Obstet Gynaecol* 1990; **97**: 1087–92.
19 Archer DF, Pickar JH, Bottiglioni F. Bleeding patterns in postmenopausal women taking continuous combined or sequential regimens of conjugated oestrogens with medroxyprogesterone acetate. *Obstet Gynecol* 1994; **83**: 686–92.
20 Benedek-Jaszmann LJ. Long term placebo—controlled efficacy and study of ORG OD 14 in climacteric women. *Maturitas* 1987; **Suppl 1**: 25–33.
21 Rymer J, Chapman M, Fogelman I. Effect of tibolone on postmenopausal bone loss. *Osteoporosis Int* 1994; **4**: 314–9.
22 Suhonen SP, Allonen HO, Lahtenmaki P. Sustained release oestradiol implants and a levonorgestrel-releasing intrauterine device in hormone replacement therapy. *Am J Obstet Gynecol* 1995; **172**: 562–7.